N. Brill

Cash's Textbook of Medical Conditions for Physiotherapists

other books in the series edited by Joan E. Cash

NEUROLOGY FOR PHYSIOTHERAPISTS

other books in the series edited by Patricia A. Downie

CASH'S TEXTBOOK OF CHEST, HEART AND VASCULAR
DISORDERS FOR PHYSIOTHERAPISTS

CASH'S TEXTBOOK OF PHYSIOTHERAPY IN SOME
SURGICAL CONDITIONS

by Patricia A. Downie

CANCER REHABILITATION
An Introduction for Physiotherapists and the Allied Professions

CASH'S TEXTBOOK OF MEDICAL CONDITIONS FOR PHYSIOTHERAPISTS

edited by
PATRICIA A. DOWNIE F.C.S.P.

FABER & FABER • London and Boston

First published in 1951
by Faber and Faber Limited
3 Queen Square London WC1
Reprinted 1951 and 1954
Second edition 1957
Reprinted 1959 and 1962
Third edition 1965
Reprinted 1968
Fourth edition 1971
Reprinted 1973 and 1975
Fifth edition 1976
Sixth edition 1979
Printed in Great Britain by
Cox & Wyman Limited
London, Fakenham and Reading
All rights reserved

© *1979 Faber and Faber*

British Library Cataloguing in Publication Data

Cash's textbook of medical conditions for
    physiotherapists. – 6th ed.
  1. Pathology   2. Physical therapy
  I. Downie, Patricia A   II. Textbook of medical
  conditions for physiotherapists
  616'.002'4616   RB111

ISBN 0–571–04991–5

Contents

Illustrations

PLATES

FIGURES

List of Contributors

MRS. J. M. ABERY, M.C.S.P.
Formerly Senior Physiotherapist, Rheumatology Unit
The Nuffield Orthopaedic Centre, Oxford

MISS S. BOARDMAN, M.C.S.P.
Senior Physiotherapist, Regional Plastic Surgery Centre
Mount Vernon Hospital, Northwood

MISS P. A. DOWNIE, F.C.S.P.
Nursing and Medical Editor
Faber and Faber, London

MISS J. HICKLING, M.C.S.P.
Superintendent Physiotherapist i/c Manipulation Unit
St. Thomas's Hospital, London

MISS B. V. JONES, M.C.S.P., M.A., DIP.T.P.
Principal, the School of Physiotherapy
University College and Mater Misericordiae Hospital, Dublin 7

MISS B. KENNEDY, M.C.S.P.
Superintendent Physiotherapist, the Paediatric Department
St. George's Hospital, London

MISS C. M. MARSHALL, M.C.S.P., DIP.T.P.
Assistant Principal, the School of Physiotherapy
Queen Elizabeth Medical Centre, Birmingham

DR A. G. MOWAT, M.B., F.R.C.P. (ED.)
Clinical Lecturer in Rheumatology, University of Oxford;
Consultant Rheumatologist, the Nuffield Orthopaedic Centre,
Oxford

J. R. PEPPER ESQ., M.A., F.R.C.S.
Senior Registrar, Thoracic Unit
Guy's Hospital, London

MISS J. M. PIERCY, M.C.S.P., DIP.T.P., DIP.PHYS.ED.
Principal, the School of Physiotherapy
The London Hospital, London

C. P. ROBERTS ESQ., M.C.S.P.
Senior Physiotherapist, Rheumatology Unit
The Nuffield Orthopaedic Centre, Oxford

MISS P. M. WALKER, M.C.S.P.
Superintendent Physiotherapist
Harefield and Mount Vernon Hospitals, Northwood

Foreword to the First Edition

by the late F. D. HOWITT, c.v.o., m.a., m.d., f.r.c.p.
Physician, with charge of Physical Medicine, Middlesex Hospital
Honorary Consultant in Physical Medicine to the Army
Senior Physician to the Arthur Stanley Institute for Rheumatic Diseases

It gives me particular pleasure to write a short foreword to this book, partly because I have read it with great interest, and partly because I am convinced that it supplies a long felt need.

The face of medicine in this country has changed considerably in recent years, mainly as the result of dire necessity imposed upon us by two World Wars. It has become less departmentalised, and has assumed a more purposeful character. We have come to realise that the achievement and maintenance of health, the conduct of serious disease and injury, and the rehabilitation and revocation of disabled persons are, none of them, a one man job. Success can only be achieved by teamwork, and in this team there are no two members more important than the doctor and the physiotherapist. Each has his separate function to fulfil, yet neither can fulfil it adequately unless he works in harmony with the other.

I suspect that Miss Cash had some difficulty in selecting the title for her book. It would manifestly be an impertinence for a doctor to write a textbook on physiotherapy for doctors, although there is great need for such a work. For it is most important that before prescribing the various forms of physical treatment, a medical man should be fully conversant with their uses and abuses, actions and reactions, indications and contra-indications. He should also realise the difficulties which beset the physiotherapist, when faced with an incorrect or inadequate prescription. It would be equally presumptuous for a physiotherapist to attempt to write a textbook on medicine for physiotherapists. Yet it is vital that the physiotherapist should appreciate the problems which the doctor has to face when assessing the likely value of physiotherapy in conjunction with other medical measures; its effect upon the constitutional and psychological condition of the patient; its prospects and sometimes its dangers. All physical treatments, whether preventive, corrective or remedial should be welded into a general and organised scheme. These are the points which Miss Cash has so admirably stressed from the viewpoint of the physiotherapist.

The author has aimed at simplicity, both in the general layout and in the description of the various medical conditions. The rationale for treatment has been fully explained in each instance, and there is a refreshing freedom from extravagant claims. It is up to date, and should serve equally as a work of reference for the qualified physiotherapist and for the senior student preparing for her diploma.

Frank Howitt

Preface to the Sixth Edition

For more than a quarter of a century Joan Cash has led the field in physiotherapy textbooks. Now, she has relinquished her editorial seat to one who was approaching her final examinations when the very first edition of this book was about to be published. In the intervening years there have been great advances in the field of physiotherapy; obscure and dubious treatments have been allowed to lapse and new ideas propagated. What is much more important is that physiotherapists are now questioning the value of treatments and no longer do they meekly obey the prescription! This does not mean that treatment is given without the doctor's directive; rather does it mean that physiotherapists work with the doctors and others in the team, to provide the best treatment available for the particular patient.

I have tried to blend some old with some new; to maintain a continuity with the familiar and at the same time to move into new areas. For this reason I have offered a chapter on the role of physiotherapy with the dying; this is an important area and allows full scope to the ingenuity of the physiotherapist while at the same time allowing her the privilege of real personal patient contact at a time of life when human contact is so often desperately needed.

I have included again a chapter on Cardiac Arrest. This is such an important fact that this particular chapter will now be included in all the textbooks in this series.

I am particularly grateful to Dr. Alastair Mowat for his help and guidance and overall editing of the chapters on rheumatology. To all the contributors I offer my thanks; it is they who have made the book; I as editor, merely put it together in a rational manner!

Once again Audrey Besterman has used her skill to produce the line drawings and together with the many X-rays and photographs I hope that physiotherapists will continue to find this textbook a clear guide to treatment principles. I would welcome suggestions for future editions, so reader, do please write and offer them!

P. A. D.
London, 1979

Chapter 1

Inflammation and Healing

revised by J. M. PIERCY, M.C.S.P., DIP.T.P., DIP. PHYS. ED.

Inflammation is the protective or defensive mechanism that occurs in the living tissue as a result of injury. It is a series of changes affecting vessels and cells surrounding the affected area. If the injury has been so severe as to cause destruction of tissue (necrosis) then the inflammatory reaction will occur in the surrounding area which has been less severely injured. The inflammation serves a two fold purpose:

a) removal of the irritant, debris and dead cells
b) preparation of the way for repair

Inflammatory reactions may be suppressed by cytotoxic drugs or immuno-suppressors and in such cases factors which would normally be trivial with ordinary reactions can become fatal.

ACUTE INFLAMMATION

Causes

There are a large number of factors which can cause the inflammatory reaction and they can be listed under the following headings:

a) Physical – thermal, mechanical, irradiation
b) Chemical – acids and alkalis, body fluids which escape into tissues (bile, urine), metabolic products of bacteria (toxins)
c) Intra-cellular replication of viruses
d) Hypersensitivity reactions such as reaction of antibody to antigenic material
e) Necrosis of tissue resulting in inflammation in surrounding area

Changes of Inflammation

Whatever the causes of inflammation, the reaction follows a basic pattern (Fig. 1/1). However, the appearance of the tissue will depend on the type of tissue affected, the nature of the irritant and the duration. The reaction may be acute, subacute or chronic. An inflammatory lesion is indicated by the suffix '*itis*' (tonsillitis, appendicitis).

The basic pattern of changes concern a) vascular, b) surrounding tissues and c) the lymph flow.

VASCULAR

The initial change may be observed in relation to superficial vessels, as a whitening of the skin. This is a momentary vaso-constriction caused by the irritant and is quickly followed by the main inflammatory changes designed to deal with the injury. The first of these changes is a relaxation of the circular muscle of the arterioles which may be brought about by a chemical mediator and possibly by the axon reflex. Whether it is one or both of these is still uncertain, although many authorities favour the chemical mediator in direct relation to the irritant. However, it may be that the axon reflex produces the more widespread flare noticed by Lewis in the 'triple response'.

Accompanying the relaxation of the arterioles there is an engorgement of the capillaries and post-capillary venules as the result of the increased blood flow (active hyperaemia). This active hyperaemia is followed by a slowing of the blood flow which results from a number of factors. There is an inflammatory exudate into the surrounding tissues which increases the viscosity of the blood in the area and thus offers more resistance to flow. The viscosity is also increased by the red cells clinging together (rouleaux). The leucocytes tend to adhere to the walls of the post-capillary venules and further hinder blood flow. In some instances there may be a temporary stasis and clotting may occur.

The inflammatory exudate is composed of a protein rich plasma which differs from the normal passage of fluid into the tissues due to hydrostatic pressure which is called transudation. The passage of proteins is accompanied by a relatively greater quantity of fluid than in normal plasma and this further increases the viscosity of the blood. There is usually an axial flow in the blood vessels with the cells and plasma lying centrally and only plasma peripherally. However, as the flow of blood slows down, the larger white cells tend to fall towards the periphery (margination) while the red cells maintain an axial flow and form rouleaux. The leucocytes (polymorphonuclear leucocytes and

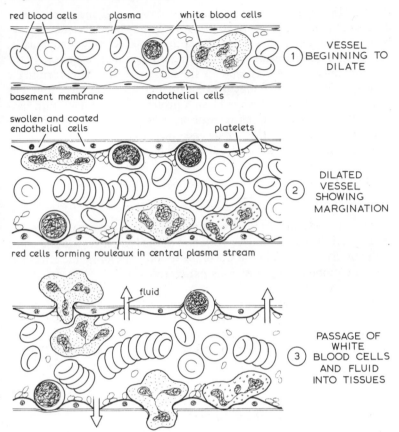

red blood cells   plasma   white blood cells

VESSEL
(1) BEGINNING TO
DILATE

basement membrane   endothelial cells

swollen and coated
endothelial cells   platelets

DILATED
(2) VESSEL
SHOWING
MARGINATION

red cells forming rouleaux in central plasma stream

fluid

PASSAGE OF
WHITE
(3) BLOOD CELLS
AND FLUID
INTO TISSUES

Fig. 1/1 A diagrammatic representation of the vascular changes which occur in inflammation

monocytes) which have adhered to the endothelial wall tend to pass out into the tissue spaces by an active process of emigration. This process occurs mainly in the venules, and the leucocytes thrust pseudopodia through the gaps in the endothelial cells and then squeeze through into the tissues. It is thought that this may be the result of chemical attraction due to a chemical mediator produced at the site of injury (chemotaxis). Some of the red cells may also pass into the tissue spaces (diapedesis).

SURROUNDING TISSUES

As already stated, there is an exudation of fluid from the vessels into the tissues and this may serve a number of purposes. The increase of fluid to the infected tissue dilutes the toxins and may prevent or diminish further tissue damage. It helps to carry bacteria and toxins to lymph vessels and nodes where the antigenic effect may further assist the defence mechanisms by producing an immune response. If the inflammatory exudate is rich in fibrinogen it may clot forming a network of fibrin which may prevent further spread of infection. The inflammatory exudate brings plasma proteins into contact with bacteria. If the plasma contains antibodies which will react with the infecting organisms they may be destroyed and removed by phagocytosis. If the ground substance of the tissues is a gel, this changes to a fluid thus preventing an early rise in tissue tension. There is a proliferation of connective tissue cells.

LYMPH FLOW

The tissues become swollen with the increased quantity of fluid in inflammation and this causes a dilation of the lymph vessels and some of the fluid escapes from the site of the lesion. The antigenic effect has been mentioned in the previous paragraph.

Although the basic changes are similar for all tissues, there are differences according to the type of tissue. For example, in mucous membrane there is an increased production of mucus which may become muco-purulent depending on the causative factor. Similar reactions will occur with serous secreting membranes.

Signs and Symptoms of Inflammation

Inflammation is characterised locally by redness, heat, pain, swelling and loss of function. In some circumstances, such as bacterial or viral infection, there may be general signs of fever with a rise of temperature, respiration and pulse rate. The presence and severity of these signs depend upon the type and degree of injury to the tissues and the efficiency of the body's defence mechanism in that area.

REDNESS

This is due to the vascular changes and can be observed if the skin is stroked firmly with a hard object. First there is a white line due to the momentary vaso-constriction. This is followed by a red line and finally a more widespread red area or 'flare' which is due to the relaxation of the arterioles and filling of the capillaries and post-capillary venules. A wheal then develops as a result of the fluid passing into the tissue spaces.

HEAT

The increased flow of blood resulting from the dilatation of vessels may cause a local increase of temperature. This can occur in superficial tissue where the temperature may be lower than the blood because of contact with the external environment.

PAIN

This is partly due to the tensions created in the tissues by the exudate. If the space is small the pressure on the nerve endings will be greater. Pain may also be due to an increased concentration of hydrogen ions or the chemical substances released by the damaged tissue.

SWELLING

The inflammatory exudate accumulates in the area resulting in swelling. The amount of swelling depends on the severity of the inflammation, the tensions of the particular tissues and the extent to which the fluid can drain away. It may also depend on the type of tissue involved.

LOSS OF FUNCTION

Inflammation will upset the function of the tissues, and the extent of this will depend on several factors. Pain, particularly in relation to muscle and joints, will limit movement and there may be reflex inhibition of muscle action. Swelling around a joint will limit movement apart from the resulting pain. Depending on the tissues involved, the inflammation may either alter or impede the function. If mucus secreting epithelium is inflamed the secretion of mucus is increased as in the common cold.

Physiotherapy

Inflammation is generally a protective mechanism and so physiotherapy would normally be used following the acute phase to assist in regaining function if there has been a loss or limitation of movement. However, if the inflammation is due to physical trauma as in acute sprain of the ankle or rupture of some muscle fibres, it may be helpful to use physiotherapeutic methods at an earlier stage.

FURTHER STAGES FOLLOWING ACUTE INFLAMMATION

Resolution

If the inflammatory agent is very mild the damaged cells and the exudate will be quickly removed and the area will rapidly return to normal. This is known as resolution. A more severe injury, provided it is not accompanied by much tissue destruction, should also resolve but the process will take a little longer, possibly up to several weeks. This return to normal occurs in the following way:

a) *Removal of excess fluid*. Most of the excess fluid drains away via the lymphatics. Some of the fluid will flow back into the capillaries as the vessels return to their normal permeability and the balance of hydrostatic pressure and osmotic pressure between the tissue fluid and plasma is restored.

b) *Removal of cellular debris and damaged phagocytes*. Debris may be digested by phagocytes or enzymes in the exudate. Some debris is carried in the lymph stream to the nodes where it is dealt with by the cells lining the sinuses.

c) *Undamaged polymorphs*. These pass back into the blood and lymph streams and macrophages wander back into the surrounding connective tissues.

Suppuration

This occurs as a result of a pyogenic bacterial infection which leads to necrosis of tissue and formation of pus. It can also occur in body cavities such as the pleural space, peritoneum or joint without involving necrosis of tissue. The toxins produced by the bacteria cause necrosis of tissue which is then digested by the polymorph enzymes leaving a space filled with pus (abscess). Pus comprises an inflammatory exudate containing living and dead polymorphs, bacteria, necrotic tissue, and fibrin. This is creamy in colour and consistency and sticky due to DNA released from the dead polymorphs.

The formation of an abscess tends to lead to an increase of bacteria and spread of infection for the following reasons: exudate from the inflammatory reaction flows into lymphatic vessels but in an abscess there is inadequate drainage and exudate tends to become stagnant. There is an increase of polymorphs into the cavity and with the exudate this increases the pressure. The exudate in the cavity is an ideal medium for the growth of bacteria and liberation of toxins which then cause necrosis of surrounding tissue. Because of the increased pressure, pus from the abscess tends to extend into surrounding tissues where there is least resistance.

CHRONIC INFLAMMATION

This type of inflammation is characterised by the proliferation of tissue cells to give fibrous tissue; this contrasts with the exudative changes of acute inflammation. Chronic inflammation may be secondary to acute inflammation when the body's defence is not sufficient to allow resolution and there is persistent low grade irritation.

Primary chronic inflammation may be produced by the same factors which produce acute inflammation but the injury or irritant produces a mild reaction. This may be due to the nature of the irritant, the dosage, the state of the body's defence and part of the body affected. Certain bacterial and fungal infections produce a chronic inflammation, e.g. tubercle bacillus and syphilis. Some dusts or chemicals produce irritation of the lungs resulting in chronic bronchitis, asbestosis or similar conditions. Repetitive minor trauma may result in chronic inflammation as in a sprained ankle.

Changes

The changes are a mixture of the vascular and proliferative changes of acute inflammation – the attempt to clear the debris and the micro-organisms and the processes of healing. This is the state in which inflammation and healing are going on at the same time.

In many cases of chronic inflammation there is extensive exudation of protein rich fluid leading to the production of considerable quantities of fibrin. This is particularly seen in chronic, suppurative inflammation and inflammation of serous sacs. Many cells are present in the area including large quantities of macrophages which may have fused to form giant cells. These cells soften and remove the dead cells and debris.

Lymphocytes and plasma cells are also found in great numbers. The function of the latter cells is uncertain but they are a feature of the granulation tissue in chronic inflammation. Endothelial cells are also present forming new capillaries. These are especially noticeable in the lining of chronic abscess cavities and they break down readily leading to haemorrhage.

Fibroblasts are present in large numbers and lay down the collagen which produces a large quantity of fibrous tissue. If the cells of the chronically inflamed tissue can divide, then regeneration occurs. Quite often there is excessive production of new cells, which is particularly noticeable in epithelial tissues.

Signs and Symptoms

These will depend on the area involved but generally lead to impaired function as a result of the formation and shrinkage of fibrous tissue. Adhesions may form in relation to ligaments around joints and will restrict movement; tubes and orifices may be affected leading to stenosis e.g. the mitral valve in chronic endocarditis or the small intestine in regional ileitis. It can lead to reduction of elasticity in tubes as in chronic bronchitis.

Physiotherapy

This will depend on the cause and the tissues affected.

HEALING

In the floor of any open and healing wound tiny raised red dots can be clearly seen. To this tissue the term *granulation tissue* has been applied. The name originates from the Latin *granum*, a seed or granule. Each dot or granule consists of new blood vessels, macrophages, fibroblasts and other cells.

No matter what body tissue is damaged, healing begins with the formation of granulation tissue. The final result may differ depending upon whether the parenchymal cells are capable of mitotic division or not. The cells of some tissues such as epithelium, bone marrow, lymph glands and the spleen continue to divide throughout life. Such tissues have great powers of regeneration. Some cells, e.g. the cells of the liver, have the power to divide but only do so if the need arises. On the other hand, nerve and muscle cells have no power to reproduce themselves and in this case granulation tissue will eventually be converted into scar tissue.

Regeneration is the replacement of lost tissue by similar tissue. *Repair* is replacement by scar tissue when the cells of the damaged organ or tissue are unable to divide.

Repair

The process of repair is best understood in the healing of open wounds but the same changes will occur in all other areas of the body where the parenchymal cells are not capable of reproducing the original tissue.

Healing of Skin Wounds

A wound where there is little tissue loss and no infection may heal by first intention (primary union). If there is a greater degree of tissue destruction then healing may occur by second intention (secondary union).

HEALING BY FIRST INTENTION

This should occur following a clean cut or surgical incision and follows a basic pattern (Fig. 1/2):

a) *Blood clot.* Blood escaping from cut vessels clots on the surface and fills the gap between the edges of the wound. This serves as an adhesive and protective cover.

b) *Inflammatory reaction.* This is mild and occurs during the first twenty-four hours resulting in exudation of fluid and invasion of the site by macrophages which ingest and digest fibrin, red cells and cellular debris.

c) *Epithelial cells.* Within twenty-four hours the squamous epithelium bridges the gap and is followed by hypertrophy of all the layers of the skin adjacent to the wound. The epithelial cells may extend down into the dermis but are later removed.

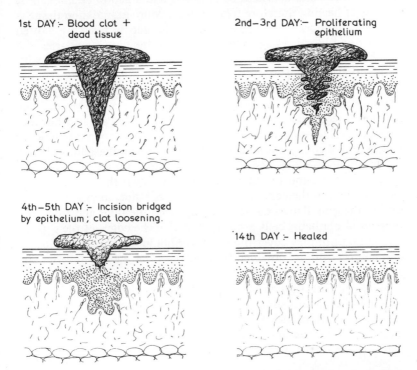

1st DAY :- Blood clot + dead tissue

2nd–3rd DAY:– Proliferating epithelium

4th–5th DAY :- Incision bridged by epithelium ; clot loosening.

14th DAY :- Healed

Fig. 1/2 A diagrammatic representation to show the stages in primary wound healing

d) *Dermis and subcutaneous tissue.* There is a proliferation of new blood vessels and fibroblasts leading to the formation of granulation tissue. Vascular sprouts extend into the wound and unite to form a vascular network and at the same time the lymphatic channels are also re-established.

e) *Fibrous tissue proliferation.* Fibroblasts proliferate and move into the area and within four to five days mature collagen fibres are produced and probably unite the cut edges of the incision from about the end of the first week.

The strength of the newly formed skin is nearly normal by about fourteen days and continues to develop slowly over the next few weeks. The normal skin formed in this manner is devoid of hair follicles, sweat and sebaceous glands which cannot reproduce.

Healing by Second Intention

There is no real difference in the healing process except that there is necrotic tissue and debris to be removed and a gap to be filled. The process of healing therefore takes longer. More granulation tissue is formed and more scar tissue results. The gap is filled by clotted exudate and blood. Phagocytic cells invade the clot. Capillaries and fibroblasts grow in from the sides and floor of the wound, filling it with granulation tissue.

If the cells of the damaged tissue can divide, new cells infiltrate the granulation tissue, but if they cannot, the tissue becomes increasingly fibrous. The collagen fibres thicken and new layers are laid down at right angles to each other, so that eventually a tough bundle or membrane of collagen fibre is formed. Tension on these fibres seems to determine the direction in which they lie. Epithelial cells at the edges of the wound multiply and migrate down the sides into the wound between the connective tissue and the clot, forcing the latter up. As the granulation tissue grows up from the floor and sides, the tongues of epithelial cells growing down on the edges of the gap are forced up until they cover the surface. Should there be much loss of epithelium, cells are obtained from the bases of the hair follicles and sweat glands.

While all this is going on some of the new blood vessels begin to atrophy while others show such proliferation of the endothelium that their lumen is obliterated. As devascularisation and thickening increase, pale, avascular scar tissue is formed. This has a great tendency to contract, thereby deforming the surrounding tissues.

Local Factors which may Affect Healing

One of the most important of these is the vascularity of the damaged tissue. A good blood supply is necessary both for an inflammatory reaction and to support the processes of repair. Circulation varies in different tissues. Some, such as bone and muscle, are highly vascular; others, such as cartilage and ligaments, have very poor nutrition and heal less readily. When the circulation is impaired by disease, healing can be seriously affected, as can be readily seen in peripheral vascular disease. The blood supply can also be reduced by a) prolonged pressure, b) oedema and c) chronic inflammation since this is accompanied by thickening of the intima and obliteration of the lumen of the blood vessels.

● Infection will delay healing since the toxins produced by micro-organisms destroy tissue.

● Persistent irritation will cause healing to be slowed, e.g. the presence of foreign bodies.

● Continual breakdown of granulation tissue due to rough handling will delay healing. Repeated dressing of a wound will have a similar effect.

● Too early movement will sometimes delay healing if it causes further damage or destruction of granulation tissue.

The speed of healing is increased by physical measures which stimulate the circulation. Thus heat, ultraviolet light, ultrasound, and moderate exercise may all help the healing process if applied correctly.

Healing of other Soft Tissues

Healing of damaged tendons takes place in an identical way to that of other soft tissues except that tendon cells are found in the granulation tissue and very slowly regeneration will occur. If the ends of the tendon are not joined, however, union will be by fibrous tissue and the danger then is that repeated stretching due to movement will elongate the fibrous tissue, lengthening the tendon and reducing power.

In a minor injury of a muscle with rupture of individual fibres, regeneration can occur but in more severe injuries scar tissue forms. Cardiac muscle fibres have no ability to divide, consequently damage to the heart muscle is healed by fibrous tissue – an infarct is converted into fibrous tissue.

Nerve tissue within the brain and spinal cord has no power of regeneration since nerve cells cannot reproduce, and axons can only grow if there is a neurilemma. Nerve fibres in the central nervous system do not have a neurilemmal sheath. Peripheral nerves on the other hand can regenerate if the cells of origin of the axons are still intact.

Healing of Bone

Again the fundamental basis of repair of bone is by the formation of granulation tissue. The final result is, however, different for two main reasons. In the first place, bone-forming cells are available in the periosteum, endosteum and bone marrow, and in the second place, when there is hyperaemia around bone, calcium is absorbed from the bone and is in high concentration in the surrounding fluid. Thus two main essentials for bone formation – bone-forming cells and calcium, are available.

BIBLIOGRAPHY

See end of Chapter 4.

Chapter 2

Oedema

revised by J. M. PIERCY, M.C.S.P., DIP.T.P., DIP. PHYS. ED.

Oedema may be defined as the accumulation of fluid in the intercellular tissue spaces and/or the body cavities. At first excess fluid is absorbed into the cells and fibres, rendering the area firmer and heavier. When the fluid can no longer be absorbed it collects in the spaces and cavities.

Oedema can be either general or local. When excess fluid is formed in the body cavities it is sometimes specially named according to the serous cavity in which it is formed, e.g. hydrothorax, hydroperitoneum, hydropericardium.

NORMAL FORMATION AND DRAINAGE OF TISSUE FLUID

Formation

Tissue fluid is formed under the influence of three main factors: i) hydrostatic pressure, ii) osmotic pressure and iii) the permeability of the capillary walls.

HYDROSTATIC PRESSURE

The blood pressure in the capillaries is higher than the pressure of the tissue fluid, consequently water and dissolved substances diffuse through the capillary wall into the tissues.

OSMOTIC PRESSURE

The osmotic pressure of the blood is largely dependent upon the plasma proteins, particularly upon the serum albumin. The capillary wall is not normally permeable, to any extent, to the larger molecules of these proteins, though a very small amount does pass through. As a result the osmotic pressure of the capillary blood is greater than that of the tissue fluid. An attractive force is therefore exerted to withdraw the fluid from the tissue space.

PERMEABILITY OF THE CAPILLARY WALL

The capillary endothelium is permeable to certain substances and not to others. Water, glucose and salts may all pass through, provided they are in greater concentration on one side of the membrane than the other. The larger molecules of the plasma proteins cannot normally diffuse, to any extent, through the endothelial cells.

Permeability can be altered. Any factor which brings about dilatation of the capillary will also increase the capillary pore size and under these circumstances the plasma proteins may enter the tissue fluid, raising its osmotic pressure and lowering that of the blood.

Drainage

Absorption of tissue fluid occurs into the blood and lymph capillaries. Since the osmotic pressure of the blood in the capillaries is greater than that of the tissue fluid, fluid is attracted back into the capillaries. At the same time the hydrostatic pressure of the tissue fluid is greater than that within the lymph capillaries, consequently fluid flows from the inter-cellular spaces into the lymph vessels. The small quantities of proteins in the tissue fluid will pass into the lymph vessels since these are more permeable than the blood capillaries. This ensures that the osmotic pressure of the tissue fluid remains low.

A balance is kept between the fluid which is formed and that which is absorbed. Thus fluid passes into the tissues and from here into the lymph vessels and so to the lymphatic glands under the influence of hydrostatic pressure and it passes back into the blood vessels under the influence of the attractive force of the osmotic pressure of the blood.

The quantity of fluid varies with rest and exercise. Activity of the muscles brings about vasodilatation and increased formation of metabolites. Vasodilatation causes increased formation of tissue fluid, while increased metabolites may raise the osmotic pressure of the tissue fluid, so that the attractive force of the capillary blood is lessened. The stiffness which follows strenuous exercise is the result of increased fluid in the tissue spaces.

FACTORS RESPONSIBLE FOR OEDEMA

Oedema may be the result of the following changes: i) increase in hydrostatic pressure of the blood, ii) fall in osmotic pressure of the blood, iii) increased capillary permeability, iv) lymphatic obstruction, v) venous obstruction and vi) slowed rate of flow of blood and lymph (Fig. 2/1).

Increase in Hydrostatic Pressure

This will, if it is sufficiently prolonged, cause oedema. It is not the only cause, since a rise in hydrostatic pressure in the capillaries means a disturbance of the circulation with change in the endothelium and increased permeability.

A rise in hydrostatic pressure may be the result of general or local factors. If the heart fails to maintain a normal circulation, there will be congestion in the veins and hydrostatic pressure will rise in the capillaries. Increased filtration will therefore occur. An obstruction in a large vein will have exactly the same effect, though it will be localised to the area which is drained by that vein.

Fall in Osmotic Pressure

This will lessen the attracting force exerted by the blood, and fluid will tend to accumulate in the tissues. Locally it may arise because the permeability of the capillary wall is increased and plasma proteins pass into the intercellular fluid. This occurs in inflammation. A fall in the general osmotic pressure may be the effect of one type of kidney disease in which a greater quantity of plasma proteins is lost through the kidney.

The plasma proteins may also be deficient due to starvation, and in this case a nutritional oedema may develop.

Increased Capillary Permeability

Trauma or nutritional disturbances may alter the permeability of the endothelium. A capillary reacts to irritation not only by dilating but also by changes in the endothelial cells which form the vessel. A great quantity of fluid may enter the tissues as a result of this factor, both in severe lacerations and in burns.

Any factor which disturbs the nutrition of the cells will also increase their permeability. If the blood is circulating unduly slowly, it loses oxygen and gains more than the normal amount of carbon dioxide. This disturbs the physical state of the endothelium and tissue fluid increases. Oedema will therefore occur, not only following trauma but also in all cases of venous congestion.

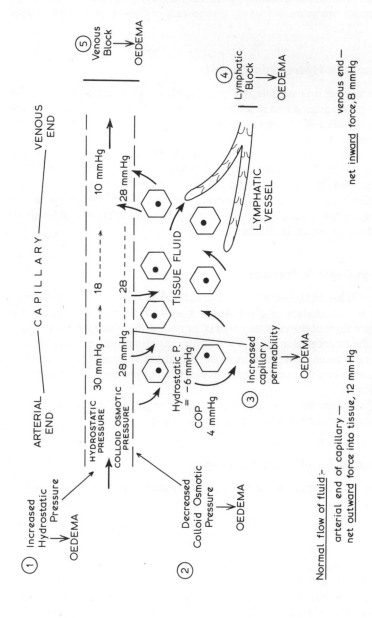

Fig. 2/1 A diagrammatic representation showing the various factors which may produce oedema

Lymphatic Obstruction

Tissue fluid may be formed normally but its drainage may be impaired because the lymph channels are blocked or because they have been removed surgically. Blocking may be due to one of the following:
a) The action of parasites such as the worm producing filariasis. This worm causes fibrosis in the vessels and glands. The oedema can be so severe in the legs and external genitalia that the name elephantiasis has been given to the condition.
b) Inflammation of the vessels and lymph glands.
c) Pressure of tumours or scar tissue.

Venous Obstruction

Obstruction to the return of venous blood to the heart will cause oedema. This can be due to right-sided heart failure, or to local obstruction arising from deep vein thrombosis or massive scar tissue formation. Overloading of the veins results in a rise in hydrostatic pressure in the venules and capillaries.

Slowed Flow of Blood and Lymph

Weak or paralysed muscles, stiff joints and poor action of the diaphragm will all reduce the venous and lymphatic return so that tissue drainage is impaired.

EFFECTS OF OEDEMA

The presence of extensive oedema is liable to set up an arterial spasm and so cause an anaemic condition of the area. Even if it fails to cause spasm it causes anaemia because, as the hydrostatic pressure of the tissue fluid rises, pressure is exerted on the capillaries and arterial inflow is retarded.

Persistent fluid in the tissue spaces interferes with the nutrition of the cells since fresh nutrient substances and gases are not available and waste products are not removed; metabolism is therefore seriously impaired and the function of the area diminished.

In the course of time, the fluid will tend to organise into fibrous tissue and the area becomes indurated. The speed with which this occurs depends upon the characteristics of the oedema fluid. If it contains a high percentage of protein it will clot readily. This condition exists when the fluid is largely the result of increased capillary permeability, and is less likely when the major factor in its formation is either raised hydrostatic pressure or low osmotic pressure. Should the fluid clot, it forms a mass foreign to the tissues and they will react by proliferation. Cells and blood vessels invade the clotted fluid and it gradually becomes converted into fibrous tissue. This may have serious effects because the fibrous tissue tends to shrink. As it shrinks it may obliterate blood vessels, so causing anaemia and gross disturbance in local nutrition. It may, if it has occurred in the peri-articular structures, cause limitation of movement in joints. Should the fluid have invaded muscles, elasticity and extensibility will be impaired. Muscular contraction may be seriously hampered by the presence of scar tissue. Should oedema occur in serous membranes, adhesions may form, causing interference with the movements of the underlying organs.

In addition to all these ill-effects, the presence of fluid distending the tissue spaces is a source of permanent discomfort and annoyance to the patient.

TYPES OF OEDEMA

Oedema occurs in many different conditions. Often therefore a special name is used to indicate the type:

General oedema: cardiac, renal, or starvation
Local oedema: traumatic, obstructive, paralytic, or oedema due to poor muscle tone and laxity of the fascia.

Cardiac Oedema

This is seen in right ventricular failure when the ventricle fails to pump out the venous blood adequately. This leads to back-pressure and congestion in the veins. If the patient is up and about, it is most marked in the lower extremities where the hydrostatic pressure is normally highest. If the patient is confined to bed it occurs in the sacral region. The oedema is worst at night when the heart is tired, and is least in the morning. Since it is mainly due to the rise in pressure in the venules and capillaries it has a low protein content and does not clot readily. If a finger is pressed over the area and then removed a depression will be left which will slowly fill as the fluid is pressed out of the tissues under the finger and then is formed again. This is known as 'pitting on pressure'.

Renal Oedema

This is most usually the result of a drop of osmotic pressure arising from increased permeability of the glomeruli to plasma proteins. The oedema is widespread and, having a low protein content, pits on pressure. It is often noticeable in the face, particularly in the lax tissues around the eyes, and is worse in the morning, tending to be dispersed by muscular action during the day.

Starvation Oedema

This is probably due to a drop in the osmotic pressure of the blood as a result of a deficiency of proteins, partly due to nutritional disturbances with loss of fat and laxity of the tissues, and partly due to decreased heart action and slowing of the circulation.

Traumatic Oedema

One of the most serious effects of extensive burns is the great loss of fluid into the tissues. This is also seen to a lesser degree in injuries such as extensive lacerations, fractures and dislocations. Various factors enter into this type of oedema.

i) Rise of local hydrostatic pressure due to the irritation of the sensory nerve endings and the release of a histamine-like substance, bringing about extensive vasodilatation and hyperaemia.

ii) Increase in the permeability of the dilated capillaries caused by the injury.

iii) Injury and possibly thrombosis of the lymphatic vessels and veins with interference to the drainage of tissue fluid.

iv) Diminished function reducing the pumping effect of muscle action and joint movement on the soft-walled vessels.

The fluid formed has a very high protein content and clots and organises readily. For this reason the final effects on the area may be serious if care is not taken.

Obstructive Oedema

This type of oedema is non-inflammatory in origin. It develops if either veins or lymphatics are obstructed. This may be the result of: i) deep venous thrombosis, ii) filariasis, iii) pressure of scars or tumours and iv) removal of lymph glands and vessels.

In a condition such as phlegmasia alba dolens (white leg), femoral thrombosis and chronic inflammation of the lymph vessels are probably both responsible. The oedema which occasionally follows radical mastectomy is an illustration of obstructive oedema which may be due to removal of lymph glands or to pressure of axillary scar tissue. The presence of fluid is mainly due to a rise in hydrostatic pressure and the fluid will have a low protein content and will clot only slowly. Nevertheless in the course of time it will organise.

Paralytic Oedema

Oedema tends to develop in the presence of extensive muscular paralysis. It is due either to paralysis of the vaso-constrictors causing widespread vasodilatation, congestion and increased filtration, or to decreased function and loss of the pumping effect normally exerted on the veins and lymphatics. If the circulation is slowed as a result of either or both of these factors, the oxygen tension of the blood will fall and the capillaries will therefore become more permeable. The fluid is likely to have a high protein content and will readily organise.

Oedema Due to Poor Muscle Tone and Laxity of Fascia

In the erect position, venous blood from the legs and abdomen has to return to the heart against the force of gravity. It would therefore have a tendency to stagnate in these regions if it were not for certain factors.

i) The deep fascia of the lower extremity is particularly strong and extensive and acts as a kind of elastic stocking to support the veins. Many of the muscles either insert directly into this fascia or send expansions to reinforce it. The fascia is affected either by prolonged recumbency or by immobilisation of the limb in a rigid support since the muscles inserting into it will become weaker and hypotonic and the fascia will become less tense.

ii) The tone of the muscles of the legs and abdominal wall plays a very important part in the prevention of 'pooling' of blood, thus any factor which causes decrease in tone may lead to venous congestion.

iii) The vasomotor mechanism causes an increase in the tone of the veins when the posture is changed from lying to standing, but if this mechanism has not been fully in use for a period of time, then when it is required it does not act as effectively as it should.

Oedema therefore tends to occur when a patient first gets up after a long period in bed, particularly if the illness has been one such as rheumatoid arthritis, in which the muscles have been directly affected and their strength and tone reduced. It will also develop when a plaster splint is removed after a prolonged period of immobilisation. In each case the inadequately constricted or supported vessels tend to dilate, venous congestion develops and excess fluid is formed, partly under the influence of a raised hydrostatic pressure and partly as a result of increased capillary permeability. The fluid will have a high protein content and will clot readily.

Idiopathic Oedema

There are a few people in whom oedema tends to develop without known cause. This is an hereditary oedema which has certain peculiar features. It affects women mainly and may involve one or both legs. No treatment appears to be effective. It causes no outstanding symptoms, but it brings about an unsightly thickening of the legs.

TREATMENT BY PHYSIOTHERAPY

The treatment of oedema depends upon the type.

General Oedema

This is rarely treated by physical measures. In these cases the treatment is medical, and if the heart lesion or the kidney disease can be alleviated, oedema is likely to disappear. Occasionally a case of cardiac oedema is met by the physiotherapist, when the main object is to hasten the absorption of fluid by the lymphatic vessels and so give the patient temporary relief from discomfort until such time as the production of excessive fluid ceases. This oedema will be treated on the same lines as obstructive oedema but with particular precautions owing to the cardiac condition.

Local Oedema

This type more commonly presents itself for physical treatment and a careful consideration of its cause must first be made.

TRAUMATIC OEDEMA

When trauma is extensive some oedema is almost inevitable. The main principle of treatment is the prevention of organisation into fibrous tissue. Efforts must be made to:

i) Decrease the formation of the tissue fluid by rest and firm support.

ii) Speed its absorption by encouraging its movement into areas in which the veins and lymphatics have not been damaged, and speed the flow of venous blood and lymph in these regions. Such measures as superficial heat and massage to the region proximal to the injury will assist.

iii) Keep the fluid moving so that it cannot clot, by elevation of the limb and rhythmic muscle contraction to press the fluid out of the tissue spaces. If muscle contractions are difficult to obtain, minimal faradic contractions may be used temporarily.

In nearly every case functional use of the limb can be encouraged early, so stimulating the tissue drainage and preventing organisation.

OBSTRUCTIVE OEDEMA

The excess fluid in this case is the result of obstruction in the venous or lymph drainage or in both. Whether the oedema will subside will depend upon how well the unobstructed vessels will dilate to do the work of the obstructed ones. The principle underlying the use of physical means is the attempt to encourage the development of a good collateral circulation. Any measures which press the fluid out of the tissue spaces and force it proximally are likely to assist, e.g.

i) With the limb elevated the fluid should be mechanically pushed on by slow, deep effleurage and vigorous active movements which press the fluid on in the veins and lymphatics.

ii) Strong muscle contractions followed by relaxation.

iii) If i) is not effective and muscle contractions not possible, faradism under pressure might prove helpful.

iv) A firm support to prevent accumulation of fluid. A one-way stretch elastic bandage must be worn and it is the physiotherapist's duty to teach the patient how and when to apply it and to give instructions about washing the bandage and its replacement when necessary.

In these cases of obstructive oedema the condition is sometimes a long-standing one and some of the tissue fluid may have organised into firm fibrous tissue which by pressure has further impeded the circulation. If these areas of induration are localised such as may be seen around gravitational ulcers, an attempt may be made to soften the fibrous tissue by the use of ultrasound and deep finger kneadings.

The most important part of the physical treatment is to teach the patient that the best way to reduce and prevent recurrence of swelling is active use of the limb while wearing a firm support. Thus walking and active exercises in the support are essential, but standing and sitting with the limb dependent are to be avoided.

PARALYTIC OEDEMA

Since the excess fluid is the result of vasodilatation and lack of use, it is difficult to prevent its formation. Continual dispersal of the fluid and movement to prevent clotting are therefore essential. Unlike traumatic oedema this cannot be carried out by the use of rhythmic contractions and active movements. Passive means must be used:

i) Elevation of the part.

ii) Passive movements of joints.

iii) Artificial exercise of the paralysed muscles by means of the interrupted direct current will exert a pumping effect on the veins and lymphatics and will keep the tissue fluid moving.

iv) Light massage is sometimes effective in dispersing the fluid into regions not affected by the paralysis, but care must be taken not to increase the paralytic vasodilatation nor to bruise or stretch the atonic muscle fibres.

OEDEMA DUE TO POOR MUSCLE TONE AND LAXITY OF THE FASCIA

Since the oedema is the result of lack of muscle tone and poor condition of fascia, the principle of treatment by physiotherapy is to bring back to normal the strength and tone of the musculature. This can be carried out by the use of maximal resisted exercises. While this is being done, constant seeping of fluid into the tissues should be lessened by repeated elevation of the limb and by firm pressure using elastic bandages. Any fluid which forms must not be allowed to organise, and measures such as those used in obstructive oedema are of value.

In all cases of oedema it is worth noting that the vessels in the region of the oedema should not be encouraged to dilate since this results in increased filtration of fluid. Dilatation of vessels which are not always patent is, however, desirable in areas proximal to the oedema. For this reason it is wiser to avoid the use of heat directly over the area. The immersion of an oedematous hand or foot in hot paraffin wax usually increases the tension in the tissues. If, due to oedema and arterial spasm, the limb is cold and blue, heat can be given to the trunk. The limb is then indirectly warmed without increasing the oedema.

BIBLIOGRAPHY

See end of Chapter 4.

Chapter 3

Thrombosis and Embolism

revised by J. M. PIERCY, M.C.S.P., DIP.T.P., DIP. PHYS. ED.

THROMBOSIS

A thrombus is a solid body formed in the cardiovascular system from the constituents of blood. Blood platelets adhere to the lining of the vessel, thromboplastin is liberated, and fibrin is formed and deposited on the little mass of platelets. More platelets then adhere and some white and red cells are trapped in the fibrinous network. The thrombus may then build up slowly, if the blood flow is normal, or quickly if the flow is slow. If the mass forms in the heart or aorta it rarely occludes the cavity but adheres to the wall, when it is known as a mural thrombus. If it forms in smaller arteries or in veins or capillaries it may completely block the vessel, and is sometimes known as an occlusive thrombus.

If a vein is involved, stasis then occurs proximal to the thrombus and the blood therefore clots to the point at which the next tributary vein joins the affected vein. Propagation of the clot may then occur because the proximal end of the clot may present a rough surface and platelets from the incoming blood start to adhere. Clotting then develops proximally to the entry of the next tributary. Eventually a clot one or two feet long may form.

If the thrombus does not dissolve, its presence causes an inflammatory reaction in the walls of the vessel. Capillary buds and fibroblasts grow into the solid mass from the deeper layers of the vessel wall while phagocytic cells remove the cellular content. Thus the thrombus becomes firmly adherent to the vessel. At this point it is unlikely to be displaced, though the proximal clot is not thus organised and can break off.

Canalisation of the thrombus gradually occurs. Endothelial cells multiply and grow into the mass between the strands of fibrin, forming new capillaries. These may join up to form channels permeating the thrombus so that the circulation in the area is re-established.

Causes

The deposit of platelets is the main feature in thrombosis and this may occur in three circumstances, a) local injury to the endocardium or endothelium, b) stasis and turbulence of blood flow and c) alteration in the coagulability of the blood.

LOCAL INJURY TO THE ENDOCARDIUM OR ENDOTHELIUM

This causes some change, whose effect is the adherence of blood platelets. The injury may be due to:

    i) disease such as occurs in atherosclerosis

    ii) surgery and accidents

    iii) anoxia

    iv) pressure on vessels (such as may occur on the veins of the calf of the leg when a patient is unconscious)

    v) chemical irritants (accounting for the inflammation and thrombosis seen in the 'drip' leg)

    vi) rheumatic heart disease in which the valves become inflamed and platelets are deposited along the edges of the cusps

    vii) coronary heart disease – damage to the endocardium close to the myocardial infarct results in formation of a mural thrombus.

STASIS AND TURBULENCE

At normal speed of the blood flow the cellular content of the blood travels at the centre of the stream, leaving a clear zone of plasma near the walls of the vessel. With slowing of the flow and turbulence, the platelets and white cells fall out into the clear zone and are therefore more likely to adhere to the endothelium. Slowing of flow may occur in the following circumstances:

    a) If a patient is confined to bed for any length of time or if a limb has to undergo prolonged immobilisation.

    b) Congestive cardiac failure.

    c) Abnormal dilatation of arteries (as in aneurysm) or of veins (as in varicose veins), such dilatations giving rise to the slowing in blood flow and turbulence.

    d) An increase in the number of red blood cells. This tends to occur in congenital cyanotic heart disease and causes increase in the viscosity of the blood.

ALTERATION IN THE COAGULABILITY OF THE BLOOD

It is known that about the tenth day following childbirth or surgery (the time at which thrombosis seems to occur most frequently) there is a rise in the number of platelets in the bloodstream. These young platelets have a greater adhesiveness.

Site

While thrombosis can occur in any part of the cardiovascular system, the commonest site is in the veins where it is associated with congestive heart failure, immobilisation and varicose veins. It also appears to be a complication of advanced cancer and it is suggested that it is then due to the release of tissue factors from necrotic tumours which affect the coagulability of the blood (Robbins and Angell, 1971). Some authorities believe that the incidence of venous thrombosis is increased by the use of oral contraceptives.

Venous thrombosis tends to complicate surgery and childbirth because several agents are then present together. These include a rise in the number of platelets and amount of thromboplastin (the latter released from damaged tissue); slowing of blood flow due to inactivity and (in the case of high abdominal or thoracic surgery), reduced respiratory excursion. Minor damage to the endothelium of blood vessels may well occur due to pressure on the calves when the patient is unconscious.

Effects of Thrombosis

The effects of thrombosis will depend upon the vessel affected, the degree to which the mass occludes the lumen, and the state of the collateral vessels:

a) Some thrombi are dissolved, probably the result of a plasminogen activator in the endothelium.

b) Some thrombi shrink and become canalised.

c) Some may become detached and form emboli and the effects then depend upon where the embolus becomes impacted.

If collateral circulation is not rapidly established in arterial thrombosis, death of tissue occurs; the dead tissue is gradually softened by autolysins and protein-splitting enzymes, and replaced by granulation tissue from the surrounding unaffected tissue. The granulation tissue changes into fibrous tissue. Such an area is known as an infarct and its seriousness depends upon the ability of the undamaged tissue to do the work of the destroyed tissue.

EMBOLISM

An embolus is a foreign body circulating in the bloodstream. When it enters a vessel too small to allow it to pass, it becomes impacted and completely blocks the vessel, producing a state of anaemia.

Though the embolus is nearly always part or the whole of a detached thrombus, it can be a globule of fat derived from ruptured fat cells or it can be air. In the former case it is a complication of fractures in which the fat, in a liquid form, is released from the ruptured fat cells of the bone marrow and passes into the veins of the cancellous spaces. In the latter case air may enter the bloodstream and so reach the heart, where it becomes churned up with the blood, forming a frothy mass which interferes with the passage of blood through the heart.

Emboli derived from a thrombus most often enter the venous circulation and so reach the right side of the heart to become impacted in the pulmonary vessels. Emboli formed in the left side of the heart may block the coronary or cerebral vessels.

EFFECT OF EMBOLISM

Both thrombi and emboli block the vessels, but the former usually produce a gradual blocking with a state of chronic anaemia. The effect of the latter is sudden, no time having been allowed for the dilatation of collateral vessels supplying the same area. In this case the result depends upon the presence of collateral vessels and the speed with which they open up. If the embolus impacts in a small vessel with many anastomosing branches, no ill effect may occur. If it obstructs a large vessel, such as the axillary artery, the limb would rapidly become cold, pulseless, cyanotic and oedematous. But warmth and colour would gradually return since blood can reach the limb through the branches of the subclavian artery, and provided these are healthy, they will rapidly dilate. There may be some residual effects, but the health of the limb will be maintained.

Should the obstruction occur in one of the main cerebral or coronary arteries which are entirely responsible for the nutrition of one area of the brain or heart, that area of tissue must inevitably undergo necrosis and infarction occurs.

REFERENCE

Robbins, S. L., and Angell, L. M. (1971). *Basic Pathology*. W. B. Saunders & Co.

BIBLIOGRAPHY

See end of Chapter 4.

Chapter 4

Tissue Pathology

revised by J. M. PIERCY, M.C.S.P., DIP.T.P., DIP. PHYS. ED.

Alteration in the size of individual cells and fibres or of an organ as a whole is not uncommonly seen. Such alteration in size is invariably accompanied by alterations in function and in many cases, though not in all, is the result of disturbances of nutrition. For any cell or fibre to maintain its normal size once it reaches full development, it must carry out its normal function, its metabolism must continue undisturbed and its nervous connections must remain intact. It follows that disturbance of any one of these factors may cause increase or decrease in size. In addition such factors as the influence of toxins, the effect of the secretion of ductless glands and interference with the blood supply must all be considered.

ATROPHY

This is diminution in the size of tissues and may be due to either a decrease in size of cells or in numbers. If the term is applied to muscles or organs it refers to the specialised elements and not the supporting framework, although in certain cases the connective tissue may increase at the same rate or even faster than the atrophy of the special cells. This increase of interstitial structures may be explained by the fact that the atrophied cells and fibres are probably receiving and using less nutrient products and oxygen, and more are therefore available for the less specialised tissues.

Common Causes of Atrophy

DIMINISHED FUNCTION

It is often seen in limbs which have been immobilised for a period of time. This is due to impaired metabolism since decreased metabolic processes mean decreased anabolism and therefore decrease in size.

Disuse atrophy, as this type is called, is seen not only in muscles but also in other tissues which have lost their function, such as the ovaries after the menopause.

INJURIES AND DISEASE OF JOINTS

These are almost invariably accompanied by rapid and severe atrophy of the muscles acting on the affected joints. Such atrophy is often much more profound than could possibly be accounted for by disuse. The probable explanation is that either sympathetic fibres are disturbed and nutrition consequently impaired, or that reflex atrophy is the result of irritation of sensory nerve endings, and so messages pass to the spinal cord and thus to the lateral and anterior horns of grey matter, causing inhibition of activity of the cells.

CIRCULATORY DISTURBANCES

A slow progressive diminution in the lumen of the main vessels of a limb means gradual cutting down of the nutrition to all the tissues of that part and all specialised cells and fibres consequently shrink in size. Involvement of skin, muscles, joint structures and bone is seen in advanced arteriosclerosis and Buerger's disease.

CONTINUOUS PRESSURE

This is responsible for atrophy partly because it reduces the blood supply to the part and partly because it impairs function and so catabolism. The presence of a tumour is liable to lead to atrophy of the tissues on which it grows.

DISEASE OF THE LOWER MOTOR NEURONES

Atrophy will be present in all structures supplied either by the damaged neurones or by any other nerve fibres running with them. Several explanations arise for this:

a) Since no nerve impulses can reach the motor end-plates there can be no muscle tone or power of contraction and the result is abolition of catabolic processes with atrophy of muscle fibres.

b) The vaso-constrictor fibres running with the motor fibres are also liable to be involved and if this occurs, paralytic vasodilatation results in circulatory stasis and impairment of nutrition to all the structures in the region. Such atrophy is serious because it is likely to continue over a long period and will therefore be followed by degeneration of the tissues and permanent impairment of function.

Most cases of atrophy are local but a generalised atrophy is seen in chronic starvation and in fevers. In the latter case the toxins stimulate protein metabolism and a rapid wasting takes place, particularly in the muscles. It is probably also partly due to impaired digestion and absorption.

Effects of Atrophy

The primary effect is decreased function. In the case of muscular tissue power depends on the number and size of the fibres. While atrophy does not normally affect the number it does affect size, and muscle power is therefore markedly reduced. In addition atrophy may mean the loss of elasticity. This is seen in the skin and may lead to limitation of function.

HYPERTROPHY

This is an increase in the size of the specialised elements of a tissue. Increase in the quantity of the connective tissues, such as in some types of muscular dystrophy, is not true hypertrophy. The change in size is due to increased functional demands or overactivity of the ductless glands. Hypertrophy may be physiological or pathological.

Physiological hypertrophy is not associated with disease. It is well illustrated in the case of the pregnant uterus or in the muscles of the athlete. Muscles in either case are called upon to do extra work and the effect is hypertrophy.

Pathological hypertrophy, as its name implies, is associated with disease. An example of such an occurrence is hypertrophy of the heart – stenosis of the mitral valve hinders the flow of blood from the left atrium and the effect is an increase in the breadth and length of the muscle fibres of the atrium. A similar hypertrophy may be seen in the involuntary muscular coat of the stomach when there is stenosis of the pyloric sphincter.

There is a limit to the amount to which any cell can hypertrophy and when this point is reached there is either hyperplasia or the functional demand fails to be met.

Pathological hypertrophy is sometimes compensatory. One group of cells and fibres enlarges to take over the work which should be done by damaged or lost tissue. This may be seen in one lobe of a lung when the other lobes have been removed, or in one kidney when the other becomes diseased and fails to function.

Hyperfunction of the pituitary gland in the adult leads to hypertrophy in the form of enlargement of the girth of the bones and thickening of the connective tissues throughout the body.

Effects of Hypertrophy

With the exception of the last mentioned type of hypertrophy, increased size means greater function. Hypertrophied muscles have always greater power than normal muscles, provided that it is the whole muscle which is hypertrophied and not only a few groups of its fibres.

HYPOPLASIA AND HYPERPLASIA

Hypoplasia and hyperplasia most commonly occur before the tissues have reached maturity and are then developmental defects, often of unknown origin.

Hypoplasia means a decreased number of cells or fibres and may be the result of disturbance of the ductless glands controlling growth and development, such as in pituitary dwarfism.

Hyperplasia is an increase in the number of cells and fibres, either as a result of increased activity of ductless glands during the period of growth, or due to greater functional demands which cannot be entirely met by hypertrophy. Hyperplasia of bone marrow very readily occurs on a demand for increased blood; division of liver cells may cause hyperplasia of the liver if a section of that organ is surgically removed; hyperplasia of the glandular tissue of the breast occurs in puberty and pregnancy. It is possible that some hyperplasia of cardiac muscle may take place but it is not a feature of voluntary muscle cells.

NEOPLASIA

The term neoplasia means new growth and the mass of cells comprising the tumour is known as a neoplasm.

This is too vast a subject to be dealt with fully in a textbook of this type but since the physiotherapist has to treat patients suffering from tumours, a brief description of some of the features of neoplasia has been included.

Most cells in the human body can proliferate, but their proliferation is under control as in the healing of wounds and when it is no longer needed, it ceases. In the growth of a tumour, the proliferation does not appear to be under control. The multiplication of cells continues even after the stimulus which seems to have evoked it has ceased.

Tumours originate from tissues in the body and may resemble these tissues. The only cells in the body which do not give rise to tumours are neurones, although their precursors do produce them (neuroblastoma). The new cells have certain characteristics: a) there are usually differences in the structure and relationship of the cells to one another, b) they lose the specialised functions of the cells from which they originated and appear to be mainly concerned with proliferation and c) in the case of malignant tumours, they have the power to form new masses at sites distal to their origin (primary growth) if they are carried away in the blood or lymph stream.

The general effect of neoplasia, particularly the malignant type, is to produce weakness and wasting (cachexia) of the normal tissues of the body while the tumour continues to grow. This may occur for a number of reasons such as the ability of the tumour to obtain nutritive substances at the expense of other tissues; direct interference with nutrition due to pressure on structures in the body, or reduction of food intake due to bacterial infection, or pain.

TYPES OF TUMOUR

Tumours are classified as benign or malignant according to their behaviour. Occasionally a benign tumour may become malignant but this is not common.

Benign

These tumours show a clearer resemblance to the tissue of origin than malignant tumours. They usually tend to be slow growing although one or two such as myomas of the uterus are fast growing. They form a mass at the site of origin and do not spread to other parts of the body. When the tumour forms in solid tissue it is usually enclosed in a capsule. A benign tumour does not generally affect the health of the patient unless it presses on vital structures or, if it is growing in glandular tissue when it can cause irritation and so increase secretion.

A benign epithelial tumour of surface epithelium is known as a papilloma, that of glandular tissue as an adenoma. Benign connective tissue tumours are usually named according to the tissue on which they grow: fibroma; osteoma; chondroma; lipoma; haemangioma; meningioma.

Malignant Tumours

Although these tumours arise in relation to a particular tissue, they are less well-differentiated than the benign tumours. The rate of growth is variable depending on their ability to spread, although generally they are faster growing than benign tumours. There is also a tendency to acquire increasingly abnormal characteristics as the disease advances.

The main characteristic of malignant tumours is invasion of the body tissues.

Malignant tumours may spread by infiltration when cells at the periphery of the mass move and grow into adjacent structures. Alternatively, the spread may be by means of lymphatic or blood vessels. The extent of infiltration depends on the primary site of the carcinoma. Carcinoma of the colon arises in the cells of the lining mucosa and spreads through the muscularis mucosae, submucosa and muscle coats to the peritoneum. Carcinoma of the breast may spread to the skin, underlying muscle and possibly to the trachea or aorta. Passage through the lymphatics or blood vessels forms the most common way in which malignant cells are spread to other tissues in the body thus forming metastases (secondary deposits) at a distance from the primary growth. The thin walls of the lymphatics, veins and capillaries are particularly liable to be penetrated. Little groups of cells may form emboli and are carried round in the vessels until they lodge in the capillary network of another tissue and form metastases. If such emboli are travelling in the venous circulation and enter via the thoracic or lymphatic ducts, the first capillary network will be in the lungs and so secondary growths in the lungs are common. Emboli in the portal circulation will impact in the liver causing metastases.

A malignant tumour of surface or glandular epithelium is known as a carcinoma, while if connective tissue is involved the term sarcoma is applied; thus we hear of liposarcoma, fibrosarcoma, osteogenic sarcoma. Various terms have been used for malignant tumours of lymphoid tissue, of which lymphatic leukaemia is one. All malignant tumours are cancers, this classification being used because of their characteristic spread into surrounding tissues.

Causes

The factor which leads to cells becoming neoplastic is still unknown but there is now a considerable amount of knowledge about predisposing or contributory causes of cancers. Substances which favour the development of tumours are termed carcinogens. There seem to be intrinsic and extrinsic factors concerned with the development of tumours.

INTRINSIC FACTORS

Genetic factors seem to lead to the development of certain tumours and particularly retinoblastoma. Polyposis coli and xeroderma pigmentosum are pre-disposing familial causes. It sometimes appears that there is a high incidence of a particular cancer in a family, but at present there is no evidence to suggest that it is inherited. High risk families should be screened regularly.

Malignant disease occurs in all races but the types of cancers vary. Carcinoma of the liver is rare in Europeans but common in Bantus. People whose skins are pale and who do not tan easily are more likely to develop skin cancer if they live in a hot climate where their skin is exposed to the sun.

There is also a different incidence of certain cancers according to the sex of the person. Carcinoma of the bronchus has been more common in the male than the female. At present, the numbers occurring in the female population are increasing which suggests that it was relative to smoking habits rather than the sex of the individual. Age is significant in relation to the development of tumours. The majority develop or become apparent over the age of 50 although some types can occur at any age. Sarcomas tend to develop in younger people and likewise some types of leukaemia develop in children.

EXTRINSIC FACTORS

Substances which are known to contribute to the formation of malignant tumours are known as carcinogens. There are an enormous variety of ways in which these carcinogens work and the production of a tumour may depend on the intensity and length of exposure or the interaction of various substances which are not carcinogenic on their own but are when combined. The following are examples of carcinogens:

1. *Chemical*: Hydrocarbons such as benzpyrene (active compound of soot and tar).
2. *Physical*: Radiant energy – X-rays, alpha, beta and gamma rays.

Alterations in the level of hormone secretions which cause hyperplasia of tissue may lead to the formation of a malignant growth. There is certainly a connection between oestrogen levels and the development of breast cancer and in the male a connection between hormones and prostatic carcinoma.

Over many years researchers have hoped that a virus would be found to be responsible for cancer as it might then be possible to protect people by vaccination. A number of viral producing tumours have been found in animals although the evidence for similar cases in man is not well proven.

Treatment

As the cause is unknown it is impossible to prevent the formation of a tumour although it may be possible to remove some of the pre-disposing or contributory causes such as the carcinogens. There is considerable evidence about the effect of carcinogens as seen by the dramatic rise of deaths from lung cancer which relates to the smoking habits of man. Great efforts are being made to reduce smoking by advertising the health risks. Similarly, preventive measures are being taken where carcinogens are involved in work situations. Protective clothing and masks are compulsory for all workers in asbestos indus-tries, and similar rules apply in furniture-making factories where wood dust has been found to be a cause of cancers of the nasal sinuses. These known industrial carcinogens are now listed and Acts of Parliament embody preventive measures as well as procedures for compensation should it be proved that a cancer has been caused through working with a specific substance.

The main form of treatment is still surgical excision and radiotherapy. If this is to be successful it is dependent on early diagnosis so that the malignant tumour may be removed before it spreads. This is not easy as many tumours do not have significant effects on health until they have spread. Thus early diagnosis is itself dependent on tests such as regular chest X-rays (in situations where there is a known hazard) or by mass X-ray checks available to the general public, cervical smear tests and instruction on breast self-examination.

PHYSIOTHERAPY

This is largely related to patients undergoing surgery and the treatment will depend on the particular surgical procedure. The physiotherapist may also be concerned with helping a patient who is terminally ill with cancer (see p. 328). This may involve help and advice on maintaining independence for as long as possible i.e. pro-vision of walking aids or helping to remove secretions from the chest to improve respiration.

BIBLIOGRAPHY

Boyd, William C. (1970). *Textbook of Pathology*, 8th edition. Lea and Febiger.
Muir's Textbook of Pathology. 10th edition (1976) (Ed. J. R. Anderson). Edward Arnold.
Robbins, S. L. and Angell, L. M. (1976). *Basic Pathology*, 2nd edition. W. B. Saunders Co.
Tiffany, Robert (Ed.) (1978). *Oncology for Nurses and Health Care Professions*, Vol. 1. George Allen and Unwin.
Walter, J. B. and Israel, M. S. (1974). *General Pathology*, 4th edition. Churchill Livingstone.

Chapter 5

Cardiac Arrest and Resuscitation

by J. R. PEPPER, M.A., F.R.C.S.

CARDIAC ARREST

This may be defined as a sudden cessation of a functional circulation. It is an emergency which demands prompt recognition. The absence of carotid or femoral pulses is sufficient. There is no need to listen for the heart beat or look for dilated pupils.

Aetiology

The heart arrests either in asystole or in ventricular fibrillation. Asystole is due usually to hypoxia, for whatever reason, or complete heart block. Ventricular fibrillation is commonly the result of an electrolyte imbalance e.g. hypokalaemia.

The common causes of cardiac arrest are:

1. Massive pulmonary embolus which obstructs the circulation and produces myocardial hypoxia
2. Myocardial infarction which can lead to sudden death probably due to ventricular tachycardia and fibrillation
3. Pericardial tamponade which restricts filling of the heart
4. Tension pneumothorax which produces an acute shift of the mediastinum compressing the opposite lung and the heart
5. Increased vagal tone which can occur during induction of a general anaesthetic and may lead to a cardiac arrest when associated with hypoxia and acidosis

Less common causes include anaphylactic reactions to drugs and air embolism.

RESUSCITATION

Unless the circulation can be rapidly restored, irreversible brain damage will occur within three (3) minutes. The priority therefore is to restore the circulation and ventilate the lungs.

If there is no board under the mattress the patient is transferred to the floor so that effective cardiac massage can be given. External cardiac massage in adults is applied by placing one hand over the other at the lower end of the sternum. The arms should be held straight as this is less tiring for the operator who may have to continue massage for several minutes before further help is available. A rate of massage of 60 per minute is the aim in adults; 80–90 per minute in children. In infants and small children the heart lies higher in the thorax so that the massaging hands should be placed over the mid-sternum. Care should be taken to avoid sudden compression of the abdomen as this may cause the liver to rupture.

Initially ventilation is achieved by mouth-to-mouth breathing or a face mask and Ambubag, taking care to maintain an airway. The patient should be intubated with an endotracheal tube swiftly and skilfully; until such skill is available it is safer to continue ventilation by face mask, keeping a close watch on the airway.

While this is going on, medical help will have arrived and an intravenous line and E.C.G. monitor will be set up. If the heart rhythm is ventricular fibrillation, D.C. counter-shock is given starting at 100 Joules (in adults) to restore sinus rhythm. If asystole is present, 1 in 10 000 adrenaline is injected either directly into the right ventricle through the chest wall or into a central venous line to induce ventricular fibrillation which can then be treated by D.C. shock. Sodium bicarbonate is given to correct the acidosis which invariably develops following a cardiac arrest.

The patient who has recently undergone open heart surgery is in a special situation. If after giving adrenaline and continuous external massage for one minute, there is no improvement the chest is re-opened via the recent wound. There are many recorded instances of patients surviving this procedure and leaving hospital in good health.

Once a cardiac output has been restored as shown by the return of the carotid or femoral pulses a search is made for the cause of the arrest and appropriate action taken. An anti-inflammatory steroid, dexamethasone, is generally given as prophylaxis against the development of cerebral oedema. However, the patient may slide into a state of low cardiac output which is insufficient to meet the needs of the vital organs; brain, kidneys and heart.

Low Cardiac Output

When such a state exists a vicious cycle develops (Fig. 5/1).

If this cycle is allowed to continue, cardiac arrest will inevitably recur. On an intensive care unit such a state should be recognised early from the following features:

1. Poor urine output; less than 30ml per hour in an adult
2. Cool peripheries and if the core and toe temperatures are being measured there will be an increase in the core:toe gradient
3. Mental confusion deteriorating eventually to unconsciousness
4. An increasing tendency to acidosis

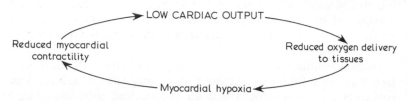

Fig. 5/1 A diagram to show the 'vicious circle' which results from a low cardiac output

Although the causes of low cardiac output are many, the basis of treatment is the same. Initially the filling pressure of the heart is examined by measuring the central venous pressure (right atrial pressure). In some cases it is useful to measure the left atrial pressure as well. Due to the relationship between cardiac output and the filling pressure of the heart as described in Starling's law of the heart, there is a critical range for optimal functioning of the heart. If the right atrial pressure is below this range which is +5 to +15mm Hg, blood, plasma or plasma expanders are given to raise the pressure. By raising the right atrial pressure to the upper limit of this range the heart is placed in the optimal physiological situation. In many instances this simple measure will suffice to restore a normal circulation.

If this is not enough, attention is directed to the state of myocardial contractility. This can be altered by the administration of synthetic catecholamines the commonest of which are isoprenaline and adrenaline. Recently dopamine has come into regular use because of its special beneficial effect on the kidneys. Other drugs in use include salbutamol and noradrenaline. A further drug has appeared recently called dobutamine. All these drugs increase the rate and force of contraction of the myocardium but in practice it is their effect on heart rate which is the limiting factor.

If after applying these measures the patient has not improved an attempt may be made to reduce the peripheral resistance. The aim of this treatment is to reduce the minimum pressure which the left ventricle has to generate in order to open the aortic valve; and thus to reduce the work done by the left ventricle. This is achieved by the administration of peripheral vasodilator drugs which reduce the sympathetic vaso-constrictor drive to arterioles. Hence, whole new vascular beds which were closed are opened up and the capacity of the circulation increases. For this reason the central venous pressure will fall and in order to maintain the heart at its optimal filling pressure, several units of blood or plasma will need to be given. This type of treatment is potentially lethal unless the central venous pressure is maintained. Examples of the drugs which are used include chlorpromazine (Largactil), phentolamine (Rogitine), nitroprusside (Nipride).

In addition the patient may be placed on intermittent positive pressure ventilation (I.P.P.V.), to reduce oxygen requirements by taking over the work of the respiratory muscles and to gain better control of the arterial oxygen tension. The acid base balance is also closely maintained and corrected when necessary.

Until recently no other routine measures were available but there are now various forms of cardiac assist devices of which the intra-aortic balloon pump is the only one in regular clinical use.

Intra-Aortic Balloon Counterpulsation

The relationship between the *supply* of oxygen to the myocardium and the *demand* by the energy processes of the myocardium for oxygen becomes critical in low cardiac output states. Drugs which increase the contractility of the myocardium and thus the cardiac output tend to do so at the expense of increased demand by the myocardium for oxygen. Such drugs may increase demand beyond the available supply and thus build up an oxygen debt. Counterpulsation provides a way of improving the ratio between supply and demand.

The concept of counterpulsation is based on the finding that myocardial oxygen consumption is dependent upon the pressure generated by the left ventricle. Counterpulsation does two things: first it increases the diastolic perfusion pressure and second it reduces the pressure against which the left ventricle contracts (a similar effect to that of the peripheral vasodilator drug).

A special balloon catheter is introduced into the descending thoracic aorta via a femoral artery. When the balloon inflates blood is displaced and the diastolic pressure in the aorta is increased. When the balloon deflates the systolic pressure is reduced and the capacity of the aorta for blood increases.

The catheter is attached to an electronically controlled actuator.

The R wave of the E.C.G. is the trigger which is picked up by the control unit. The trigger is delayed so that the balloon is inflated during diastole when the aortic valve is closed. Since the majority of coronary blood flow occurs during diastole and is dependent upon diastolic perfusion, the selective elevation of diastolic pressure by the balloon will increase coronary blood flow. Shortly before the onset of left ventricular systole the balloon is deflated. This reduces the systolic pressure against which the left ventricle ejects its blood and so reduces work and hence myocardial oxygen consumption by the left ventricle.

The counterpulsation pump is used in two clinical situations. Firstly in the operating theatre to enable a struggling heart to take on the load of the circulation and so come off cardiopulmonary bypass. Second, to assist a patient in low cardiac output, either following open heart surgery or as a means of holding a severely ill patient with coronary artery disease for a limited period before emergency coronary artery vein bypass surgery is done.

Chapter 6

Polyarthritis of Unknown Cause – I

by A. G. MOWAT, M.B., F.R.C.P. (Ed.) and J. M. ABERY,
M.C.S.P.

Introduction

Arthritis affects as many as 5 million people in the United Kingdom, a
very large majority of whom are afflicted by two quite separate diseases. Approximately 1·5 million people have rheumatoid arthritis,
although fortunately only a small proportion have serious disease or
disability, while approximately 3·5 million people suffer from various
forms of degenerative arthritis, osteoarthrosis. Although many
patients with degenerative arthritis have ceased to be wage-earners, it
has been estimated that the combined cost of lost production and
sickness payments attributable to arthritis exceeds £500 million per
annum. This far exceeds the annual cost to the nation of all strikes and
places arthritis second only to chronic bronchitis in this unattractive
'league'. These figures, although important, fail to emphasise the real
problem of arthritis, which is that the quality of the lives of these
patients is impaired by pain and disability.

Fortunately, there is a growing interest in and concern for these
patients. This is reflected in a growing public awareness of the problems of the disabled and in action by the Department of Health and
Social Security to increase the number of doctors in the field of
arthritis and to develop Demonstration Centres for the treatment of
the disabled. At the same time, increasing financial support for
research into the causes and treatment of these diseases has begun to
show important results, with the availability of new drugs, the use of
better programmes of management and the development of an excit-
ing range of new orthopaedic prostheses and appliances.

There are no general rules for the management of patients with
arthritis and an individual programme of treatment has to be planned
for each patient after careful assessment of his or her problems. These

chapters contain sufficient information for sensible programmes of management to be planned. Such management will reduce disability and improve the quality of the arthritic's life.

CLASSIFICATION OF JOINT DISEASE

POLYARTHRITIS OF UNKNOWN CAUSE

Rheumatoid arthritis
Juvenile chronic polyarthritis

POLYARTHRITIS OF UNKNOWN CAUSE

Ankylosing spondylitis
Reiter's disease
Reactive arthritis
Psoriatic arthropathy
Arthropathy of ulcerative bowel disease

A common thread of genetic influence, familial aggregation and spinal involvement runs through this group of sero-negative polyarthritides.

ARTHRITIS DUE TO INFECTION

Rheumatic fever
Septic arthritis
Gonococcal arthritis
Brucellosis
Tuberculosis
Viral arthritis
Erythema nodosum

Although the pattern of arthritis differs widely, infection or an allergic process secondary to infection is important in all the diseases in this group.

CONNECTIVE TISSUE DISEASES

Disseminated lupus erythematosus
Dermatomyositis
Scleroderma
Sjögren's syndrome
Polyarteritis nodosa
Polymyalgia rheumatica

These connective tissue diseases, most of which are rare, have an inflammatory reaction in arterioles as a common pathological basis. Important immunological abnormalities are often present. Although multi-system disease is the rule, there are prominent and often early symptoms and signs in the musculo-skeletal system and the involvement of the joints may resemble that found in rheumatoid arthritis. Most carry a poor prognosis.

CRYSTAL ARTHRITIS

Gout
Pyrophosphate arthropathy (pseudo-gout)

OTHERS

Arthritis associated with malignant disease
Arthritis associated with haemophilia
Arthritis associated with neurological disease

DEGENERATIVE ARTHRITIS

Osteoarthrosis
Spondylosis and intervertebral disc disease

NON-ARTICULAR PAIN

RHEUMATOID ARTHRITIS

Rheumatoid arthritis is a common inflammatory disease of joints, characterised by symmetrical, peripheral polyarthritis often associated with systemic features. The name rheumatoid disease may be preferred since it directs attention to the whole patient.

INCIDENCE

Rheumatoid arthritis affects some 3 per cent of the population of Great Britain. Although it was once thought only to affect populations living in temperate climates, it is now clear that the incidence of the disease is much the same the world over, but causes less disability amongst those living in warmer climates. Two-thirds of cases begin before the age of 50 but no age group is exempt. An acute onset in the eighth or ninth decade is well documented, although the disease tends to be more benign and spontaneous remissions are more common. The disease affects females to males in a ratio of 3:1.

Clearly the disease afflicts young people at the most important time of their lives, when wage-earning is at a peak and when housewives have young children to look after. It is these reasons, together with the

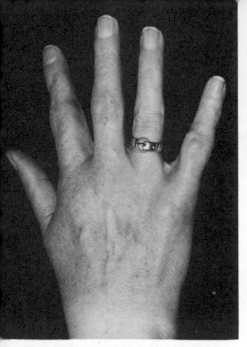

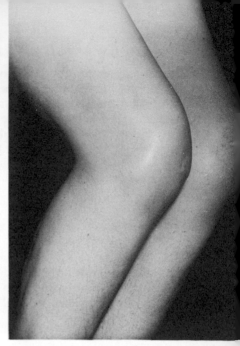

Plate 6/1 Rheumatoid arthritis of the hands, showing swelling of the metacarpophalangeal and proximal interphalangeal joints of the second, third and fifth fingers

Plate 6/2 Rheumatoid arthritis of the knees showing gross flexion deformity

chronicity of the disease, which necessitate the total management of the patient and not just of the joint disease.

Clinical Features

The disease is characteristically polyarticular and although the onset may be monarticular the spread to involve other joints, usually producing symmetrical disease, is often rapid. The small joints of the hands and feet are first affected in 70 per cent of patients, although in older patients the shoulder joint is commonly involved first. The onset is acute, with fever and constitutional symptoms in 20 per cent of patients.

The patients complain of loss of function, pain and stiffness, most characteristically in the morning. The joints and the surrounding peri-articular structures, tendons, ligaments and joint capsules are tender and swollen (Plate 6/1). Synovial proliferation and joint effusions may be marked. There is limitation of joint movement and correctable flexion deformities may follow at many joints. These flexion deformities accommodate the swollen and proliferating tissues with a reduction in pain (Plate 6/2). If the inflammatory process is unchecked further deformity and disability will result due to the progressive damage to joint cartilage, subchondral bone and peri-articular structures and to the associated muscle spasm. Flexion contracture is the common deformity in a large joint. *In the hands* more characteristic deformities such as ulnar deviation, swan neck (hyperextension at the proximal interphalangeal and flexion at the distal interphalangeal joints) and boutonnière deformities (flexion at proximal interphalangeal and hyperextension at distal interphalangeal joints) of the fingers may develop. *In the feet*, broadening of the forefoot, clawing of the toes and plantar callosities may develop. These changes are due to alterations in the intricate mechanical arrangements of the tendons, ligaments and joints.

In the knee, effusions occur early. Later, flexion, valgus and external rotational deformities develop. In early disease, use of the knee while it is distended by effusion may lead to the development of a posterior joint cyst or joint rupture. The latter mimics a deep venous thrombosis but can be easily diagnosed by arthrography. Similar cysts or rupture may occur at other joints. Although involvement of the sacro-iliac and spinal joints is uncommon, important complications can arise in the upper cervical spine.

Instability of the atlanto-axial joint with subluxation of the atlas on neck flexion is a radiological finding in 25 per cent of patients (Plates 6/3 and 6/4). They complain of pain, particularly with jolting movement, C1–2 root compression symptoms and occasionally demonstrate signs due to spinal cord compression. Although symptoms and signs are less common than the radiological findings would suggest, sudden death due to cord compression has been recorded and if surgery is planned the anaesthetist should be warned so that appropriate protective measures can be taken. Management of pain and root compression is by the use of cervical collars, but the presence of persistent symptoms or cord compression demands surgical fixation.

Tendons in synovial sheaths become involved in the same pathological process as affects the joint synovium. Tendon sheath involvement, which is usually on the flexor and extensor aspects of the hand and the forearm but occasionally around the ankle, may impair function. More extensive disease leads to tendon damage and stretching or rupture, particularly of the extensor tendons of the fingers at the wrist, may occur. Bursae in a wide variety of sites may also become inflamed. The usual sites are over the head of the first metatarsal joint ('bunion') and the olecranon.

Progressive disease causes further loss of cartilage and bone with subluxation of joints. The end result is ankylosis.

However, it must be appreciated that the progress of the disease and

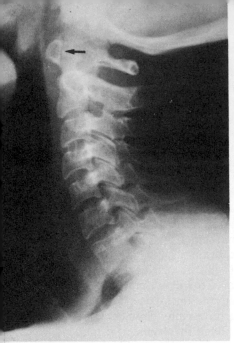
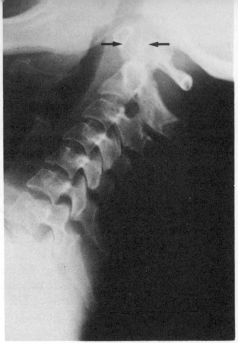

Plate 6/3 Lateral radiographic view of a rheumatoid arthritic neck taken in extension. The arrow shows the proximity of the arch of the atlas to the odontoid process

Plate 6/4 Lateral radiographic view taken in flexion of the same neck as 6/3. The arrows show the large gap between the anterior arch of the atlas and the odontoid process (the normal gap is 2–3 mm)

the ultimate damage produced by the disease varies considerably. A large proportion of patients have very mild disease which causes little or no disability or deformity and may not necessitate advice from their family doctor, let alone a hospital specialist. Others may have disease of acute onset which causes considerable pain and disability for several weeks or months but which is subsequently well-controlled by appropriate therapy and then causes little trouble. Yet others may have disease with a gradual onset which causes progressive, severe damage despite all attempts at control. Certainly natural variations in the intensity and activity of the disease are common and these tend to produce remissions or relapses lasting many months. The variability in the natural history of the disease makes a uniform description impossible and makes discussion and management of individual cases difficult.

Extra-Articular Features

Rheumatoid arthritis is a systemic disease. Loss of appetite and weight, general malaise and depression are common. A low-grade fever may be present. Generalised osteoporosis with more marked juxta-articular osteoporosis occurs and muscle wasting is prominent, around both involved and uninvolved joints. Lymph node and splenic enlargement is common. Almost all patients have some degree of anaemia due to abnormalities in iron metabolism. Oral iron therapy is of no value. The anaemia can be improved by controlling the disease or by parenteral iron therapy.

Thinning of the skin due to loss of the subcutaneous fat and connective tissues is common. Shearing stresses on the skin tend to cause bruising since the small vessels are poorly supported and patients may need to protect skin overlying bone such as the shin. Fortunately wound healing after surgical procedures is normal.

Many of the complications of rheumatoid disease can be attributed to inflammatory changes in small arteries and arterioles. These can cause small necrotic lesions at the periphery, particularly around the nail folds, and may even lead to small areas of gangrene. Such vascular changes form the basis of the neurological and pleural lesions to be described and are the cause of the rheumatoid nodule. They occur only in those with positive serological tests for rheumatoid factor. Characteristic subcutaneous nodules, present in 20 per cent of patients, develop over any pressure areas, particularly the extensor surfaces of the forearms. Their removal, unless they become infected or for mechanical reasons, is probably unwise since they frequently recur.

Nerve involvement includes mono-neuritis multiplex with involvement of one or more major nerves producing such signs as foot drop and the very serious symmetrical, peripheral neuropathy producing motor weakness and stocking and glove sensory loss, both of which are due to vasculitis of the vasa nervorum. Entrapment neuropathies are a common feature of rheumatoid disease and may be the presenting complaint. Compression of the median and posterior tibial nerves in the carpal and tarsal tunnels respectively and entrapment of the ulnar nerve at the elbow and the common peroneal nerve at the head of the fibula are well documented. Proliferation of tendon sheath or joint synovial tissue in a limited space is responsible. Carpal tunnel compression occurs in 60 per cent of patients at some time. Surgical decompression of nerves may be required.

In the chest, rheumatoid nodules may develop in the lower lung fields and be confused with a tumour. Pleurisy and pleural effusion occur but the most serious lesion is the untreatable diffuse interstitial fibrosis which leads to progressive shortness of breath.

Various inflammatory changes in the eye may impair vision and further disable the patient.

COMPLICATIONS

Amyloidosis, the term given to the deposition in tissues of an abnormal protein, is found post mortem in 20 per cent of patients with rheumatoid arthritis. It may present as renal damage with proteinuria progressing to nephrosis but comparatively few patients show any signs of amyloidosis during life. Septic arthritis superimposed upon rheumatoid arthritis will occur in 3 per cent of patients. Although the septic process, which is usually due to *Staphylococcus aureus*, may be silent, the apparent flare-up of rheumatoid arthritis in only one joint should be considered as septic arthritis until proved otherwise.

Aetiology

The cause remains unknown. It is likely, based upon evidence from human remains and paintings, that the disease appeared in its present form some 350 years ago. Although a viral aetiology remains probable, the most elaborate bacteriological studies have failed to identify a virus or other organism in the synovial fluid or tissue of even the earliest cases. It seems likely that there may be several initiating factors which are distinct from a perpetuating mechanism about which there is more general agreement. Thus, there is evidence of abnormal protein production, probably in the form of an antibody to altered tissues or proteins, which can produce a series of inflammatory reactions ending in the production of synovitis. The mechanism providing the stimulus to this antibody production is unknown but the following factors have been suggested.

A GENETIC INFLUENCE

There is a tendency for the disease to be aggregated in families. However, even though many patients carry the tissue typing antigen HLA DW4, detailed family studies have failed to provide definite evidence of genetic transmission. Certainly patients should not be allowed to become unduly concerned about the chances of their offspring developing the disease and the increased risk should not, on its own, be allowed to influence their decision to start a family.

TRAUMA

Many patients have mentioned traumatic incidents as a precipitating cause but detailed studies do not support this theory. Patients rarely receive compensation if the disease apparently develops following an industrial accident.

PSYCHOLOGICAL STRESS

Patients frequently suggest this reason but this reflects their natural desire to find an explanation for a disease which has no clear cause. It has been difficult to support this entity by statistical means except in some cases of identical twins in whom rheumatoid arthritis affected only the twin under stress.

ENVIRONMENT

Although spouses do not show an increased incidence of the disease, environmental factors probably play some part, since, for example, there is a higher incidence in urbanised Africans than in the same population remaining in primitive communities.

VASCULAR CHANGES

Alteration in the normal peripheral vascular bed, perhaps by the sympathetic nervous system, has been suggested as the primary abnormality and has been implicated to explain the striking symmetry of the arthritis in many patients.

Diagnosis

Although rheumatoid arthritis is much the commonest form of inflammatory joint disease, it is important that the diagnosis is made soundly so that appropriate treatment can be started and the implications of the disease can be explained to the patient. The American Rheumatism Association has laid down certain criteria for the diagnosis of rheumatoid arthritis:

1. Morning stiffness
2. Pain on motion or tenderness in at least one joint
3. Swelling of at least one joint
4. Swelling of another joint within three months
5. Simultaneous involvement of the same joint bilaterally but excluding the distal interphalangeal joints of the fingers
6. Subcutaneous nodules
7. Radiograph (X-ray) changes typical of rheumatoid arthritis
8. A positive test for rheumatoid factor
9. A poor mucin clot of the synovial fluid
10. Characteristic histology of the synovial membrane
11. Characteristic histology of the nodules

Criteria 1–5 must be present for six weeks. When 20 other causes of polyarthritis listed by the American Rheumatism Association have been excluded the diagnosis of rheumatoid arthritis can be considered. Classical rheumatoid arthritis requires seven and definite rheumatoid arthritis five criteria. It should be stressed that the diagnosis can be made on a clinical basis by using criteria 1–5 and that the finding of a positive test for rheumatoid factor is relatively unimportant using this list of unweighted criteria.

Laboratory Findings

Anaemia with a haemoglobin value of 11g per cent is common. The white cell count is usually normal but a rise to 10–$15 \times 10^9/1$ occurs with steroid therapy and superimposed bacterial infection. The ESR may be markedly elevated and in some patients with long-standing disease may never return to normal value. The tests for rheumatoid factor are positive in 70 per cent of cases. Positive tests are less common in those with onset of the disease late in life. It must be remembered that positive tests occur with increasing frequency in the normal population with age. Positive tests also occur in the other connective tissue diseases and in diseases in which marked changes in the serum globulins occur such as multiple myeloma, macroglobulinaemia, chronic infections and liver disease. Unaffected relatives of patients have a higher than expected incidence of positive tests.

RADIOLOGY

The sequence of radiological signs (Plates 6/5 and 6/6), of rheumatoid arthritis are:

1. Soft tissue changes around a joint due to synovitis and effusion
2. Osteoporosis
3. Periosteal reaction with new bone formation along the shaft adjacent to capsule attachments
4. Subchondral cyst formation
5. Narrowing of joint spaces due to cartilage loss
6. Loss of bone substance by erosion along the marginal areas of the joint
7. Subluxation and deformity
8. Bony ankylosis

PATHOLOGY

Inflammation of synovial tissue in joints, tendons and bursae is the essential pathological change. The thickened, oedematous, inflamed tissue produces erosions of the cartilage surface and erodes into the subchondral bone. These erosions may become larger and cystic and lead to joint destruction. Reparative changes are rarely found and the disease progresses to fibrous and occasionally bony ankylosis. Microscopically the synovium is vascular and infiltrated with lymphocytes and plasma cells which are clumped together in follicles. It must be emphasised that present pathological techniques do not allow a firm diagnosis of rheumatoid arthritis when biopsy material is examined. Very similar changes are found in many types of inflammatory joint disease.

Prognosis

One of the greatest problems arises from the variable nature of the disease and it is very difficult to give an accurate prognosis in individual cases. However, the general prognosis is better than many expect, especially when it is appreciated that follow-up studies have only been done on patients attending hospitals and special units, who inevitably have more severe disease. Follow-up studies on large numbers of patients treated by simple methods show that after 10 years 50

Plate 6/5 Radiograph of a hand with rheumatoid arthritis showing osteoporosis and cartilage and bone damage, especially in the second, third and fourth metacarpophalangeal joints and the third proximal interphalangeal joint

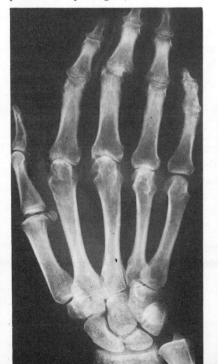

Plate 6/6 Radiograph of a hand with advanced rheumatoid arthritis, showing subluxation at the metacarpophalangeal joints and bony ankylosis at the wrist with disappearance of individual carpal bones

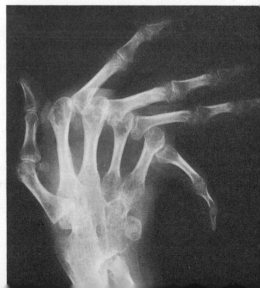

per cent will have improved and 50 per cent deteriorated. This important fact, which underlines the known tendency for the disease to remit and relapse, must be remembered when any form of therapy is being evaluated.

Earlier studies, grading such patients according to their disability showed that approximately 20 per cent had no disability; 40 per cent had moderate disability; 30 per cent had more severe disability but remained independent in the home and usefully employed; 10 per cent were dependent upon others. The disease was inactive in 25 per cent of the patients. However, these figures are no longer accurate. The increasing use of powerful disease-influencing drugs such as gold salts and penicillamine is increasing the percentage of patients with no or only moderate disability, and the increasing use of orthopaedic surgical treatment, particularly total hip replacement, is reducing the percentage of patients dependent upon others. Thus the concepts that large numbers of patients become crippled and that the disease becomes 'burnt out' are erroneous.

Factors that suggest a poor prognosis include insidious onset, unremitting disease, the presence of nodules and other vasculitic phenomena, severe systemic involvement with a high ESR and anaemia, and the presence in the serum of rheumatoid factor in large amounts. Although few patients die from rheumatoid arthritis per se, the disease reduces life expectancy by five to eight years. Death from bacterial infection and renal disease is commoner than in the general population.

MANAGEMENT

The basic principles, the use of rest, exercise, splints and walking aids and domestic and occupational factors are discussed in Chapter 9. Surgical treatment is discussed in Chapter 12 and drug therapy in Chapter 15.

JUVENILE CHRONIC POLYARTHRITIS

It is now clear that this description includes several different disease entities and it is important that these should be differentiated since they produce different problems and have different prognoses. The diagnoses are dependent upon the children being under sixteen years of age at onset and the symptoms having been present for at least three months.

1. Chronic polyarthritis with systemic features
2. Chronic polyarthritis with iridocyclitis

3. Chronic polyarthritis associated with other diseases such as psoriasis and ulcerative bowel disease
4. Juvenile rheumatoid arthritis
5. Juvenile ankylosing spondylitis

The peak age of onset of the chronic polyarticular forms is between two and four years with a second peak around puberty. Juvenile rheumatoid arthritis and ankylosing spondylitis tend to start later in childhood. In all types, monarticular arthritis, commonly involving the knee, is the usual presentation. The disease occasionally remains monarticular but in the majority becomes polyarticular with involvement of knees, hands, wrists and feet. In the chronic polyarticular forms early involvement of the hips and cervical spine is common, while with the passage of time juvenile rheumatoid arthritis and ankylosing spondylitis develop into the adult forms of these diseases with, in ankylosing spondylitis, the regression of peripheral joint symptoms.

Although the increased thickness of the articular cartilage seems to retard the appearance of erosions, unremitting disease leads to joint damage often with bony ankylosis. Increases in peri-articular vascularity, the presence of systemic disease and the use of corticosteroids may cause a variety of skeletal growth abnormalities. A small chin is one such striking abnormality. Although general malaise, loss of appetite and weight may occur in any case, more characteristic systemic signs are found in some children with polyarthritis. These are: fever; lymphadenopathy; splenomegaly; rash – a dusky pink eruption, the distribution of which may vary from hour to hour; anaemia; white cell counts up to $20 \times 10^9/1$; pericarditis; the ESR is elevated. Tests for rheumatoid factor are negative except in those children with juvenile rheumatoid arthritis.

Iridocyclitis, which is a very serious and often insidious, form of eye inflammation may occur in children from any group but is commoner in those with positive anti-nuclear tests. Certainly those with positive tests should have periodic eye examinations and the parents should be warned to seek medical advice immediately there are eye symptoms.

Girls predominate in all forms except the ankylosing spondylitic variant in which tissue typing for the presence of the HLA B27 antigen can be a useful diagnostic test.

Children with rheumatoid arthritis or ankylosing spondylitis carry the disease into adult life when it follows the typical course of the disease. Some 5 per cent of children carry the chronic polyarticular forms into adult life. Of those in whom the disease remits, 50 per cent will have no residual damage, 45 per cent will have moderate deformity and disability and 5 per cent will be severely incapacitated. A better prognosis is enjoyed by those whose disease starts in early childhood, is treated within a year of onset and whose involvement is monarticular. Juvenile chronic polyarthritis must be differentiated from rheumatic fever, viral and septic arthritis, the connective tissue diseases and the leukaemias.

Treatment

Treatment chiefly involves the proper management of the patient as a child with the provision of the necessary hospital, home and educational facilities to achieve this end. It must be realised that many of these children will eventually earn their living by 'brain' and not by 'brawn', and that in consequence the maintenance of their education, even when in hospital, is vital.

Prevention of deformity in a disease with a high remission rate is crucial. All the methods described for adult rheumatoid arthritis are of value except that sustained immobilisation in splints is inadvisable because of the tendency of joints to ankylose. Drug therapy in appropriate dosage follows similar lines. Corticosteroid therapy must be used with care because of the effect on growth. ACTH and alternate day oral steroids reduce these effects.

Surgical treatment is largely confined to reconstructive procedures. These may be carefully timed with examinations in teenagers or delayed until early adult life when the disease has remitted. Although there have been reports of the satisfactory results of synovectomy, especially in the knees, on both the local and the general disease states, the operation is not widely used. Surgical procedures are best avoided in children under the age of 6 years whose co-operation may be difficult to obtain.

BIBLIOGRAPHY

See end of Chapter 12.

Chapter 7

Polyarthritis of Unknown Cause – II

by A. G. MOWAT, M.B., F.R.C.P. (Ed.) and J. M. ABERY, M.C.S.P.

ANKYLOSING SPONDYLITIS

Ankylosing spondylitis is a chronic inflammatory disease involving chiefly the synovial diarthrodial and cartilaginous joints of the spine. Population studies suggest that the disease affects as many as one per hundred with an equal sex incidence. However, as a clinical problem, the incidence is one per thousand with a male:female ratio of at least 4:1.

Pathology

The essential abnormality is an inflammatory reaction originating in the attachment of ligaments and joint capsules to bone (an enthesopathy). The inflammatory reaction, consisting of a lymphocytic and plasma cell infiltrate and increased vascularity and fibrosis, extends to involve spinal ligaments, the outer layers of the intervertebral disc and posterior apophyseal joints. Sacro-iliac joint involvement always occurs and peripheral synovial joints may also be affected, the synovial reaction resembling that found in rheumatoid arthritis. Continuing inflammation results in calcification and subsequently ossification of ligaments and the ankylosis of joints.

Clinical Features

The disease usually begins between the ages of 16 and 40 years. The onset is gradual and initial complaints of lumbar backache and discomfort after rest may be ignored. Some patients may progress to serious deformity and ankylosis before seeking advice. However, most patients complain of backache (with radiation of the pain down

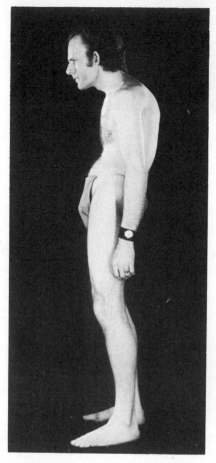

Plate 7/1 Advanced
ankylosing spondylitis
showing the spinal
deformity, flat chest and
ballooned abdomen

the back of the thighs as far as the knee) and marked stiffness especially after immobility in a car or theatre seat and for an hour or more
each morning.

Any part of the spine may be involved, although the disease usually
starts in the lumbar spine and proceeds upwards. Loss of the lumbar
spinal curve and progressive kyphosis of the remainder of the spine is
usual (Plate 7/1). The involvement of synovial costo-vertebral joints
leads to progressive reduction in chest expansion. In severe cases
respiration may be entirely diaphragmatic, leading to abdominal bal-
looning. (Thoracic girdle pain is common, while the cervical spine is
extended to allow the patient to look forward.) Any involved joint or
bony prominence may be tender and pain may be elicited by forced
movement of the sacro-iliac joints.

Although involvement of peripheral joints (most commonly the hip and shoulder) may occur in 50 per cent of patients at some time, in 10 per cent of cases synovitis of a peripheral joint or tendinitis (Achilles tendinitis, plantar fasciitis) is the presenting feature and may lead to diagnostic difficulties. Many patients will have systemic signs of the disease such as low-grade fever, anaemia and weight loss. The ESR is usually elevated but the rheumatoid factor tests are negative.

Careful measurements of all planes of spinal movement and chest expansion are valuable in the assessment and management of ankylosing spondylitis, although such measurements are now considered less valuable in the diagnosis since these measurements vary widely in the normal population and decrease with age.

The most commonly used measurements and ones that can usefully be undertaken by the physiotherapist are:

1. Occiput to wall distance with the patient standing erect with his heels against the wall and the cervical spine in the neutral position. Watch out for bending of the knees and extension of the cervical spine.
2. Chest expansion measured below the breasts and pectoral muscles.
3. Schober index of lumbar spinal flexion. Marks are placed on the skin overlying the lumbo-sacral junction which is represented by the spinal intersection of a line joining the dimples of Venus, and 10cm above this point. The distraction between these marks on full forward flexion is recorded.
4. The distance between finger tips and the floor on full forward flexion with the knees together and straight.

It is important to remember that the patient may compensate for spinal rigidity by increased hip flexion and so still be able to touch his toes. (Examination of the undressed patient avoids such errors.) Limitation of movement may be reversible if due to pain and muscle spasm.

Complication

Recurrent iritis, a painful inflammatory process in the eye, occurs in 10 per cent of cases and may occasionally be the presenting feature. Energetic treatment with local corticosteroids is required to avoid permanent visual impairment.

Atlanto-axial subluxation is common, and hence spinal cord damage may occur especially if the remainder of the spine is rigid or the neck of the unconscious or anaesthetised patient is handled carelessly. Fracture of the rigid but brittle spine occasionally occurs.

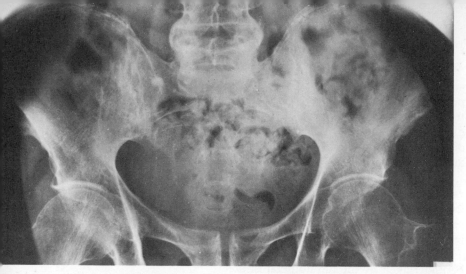

Plate 7/2 Radiograph showing ankylosis of both sacro-iliac joints in a patient with ankylosing spondylitis

Plate 7/3 Radiograph showing the typical 'bamboo spine' seen in ankylosing spondylitis. Bony bridges can be seen between the vertebral bodies

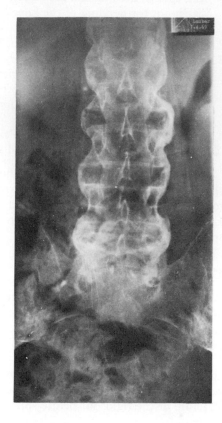

There are clear associations with psoriasis and ulcerative bowel disease (see p. 85).

Radiology

The diagnosis of ankylosing spondylitis cannot be considered unless there is evidence of bilateral sacro-iliitis. However in very early cases and in teenage patients the interpretation of the radiographs may be difficult. The sequential appearances in the posterior–anterior films are of erosive arthritis, marginal sclerosis and finally bony fusion with disappearance of the sclerosis (Plate 7/2). Spinal radiographs may show ligamentous ossification, ankylosis in apophyseal joints, the typical spinal deformity with squaring of the vertebral bodies and 'a bamboo spine'; an appearance due to new bone growth between adjacent vertebrae resulting from the changes in the intervertebral disc (Plate 7/3).

Differential diagnosis and aetiology

The diagnosis of ankylosing spondylitis is based upon the presentation of: 1) thoraco-lumbar pain and stiffness, 2) limited spinal and chest movement, 3) radiographic evidence of sacro-iliitis and 4) an elevated ESR in 75 per cent of cases. Similar findings may occur in Reiter's disease, juvenile chronic polyarthritis, psoriatic arthropathy and in the arthritis associated with ulcerative colitis and Crohn's disease, although additional features in each of these diseases usually allow the correct diagnosis to be made. All these diseases may be associated with iritis, and the nature of this curious link between sacro-iliac joint disease and the eye is unexplained. These diseases are further linked by the finding of an increased familial aggregation and the fact that the tests for rheumatoid factor are negative. Genetic rather than environmental factors are likely to be important in these diseases.

In 1973 the genetic influence was confirmed by the finding that 95 per cent of patients with ankylosing spondylitis carried the tissue antigen HLA B27. However, the relative rarity of the disease, and the presence of the antigen in 6 to 8 per cent of the normal population, means that this expensive test has little value in the assessment of young men with backache. However, the test is useful in the evaluation of atypical cases and, as discussed earlier, is useful in identifying a group of male children with juvenile chronic polyarthritis who will go on to develop ankylosing spondylitis. Children of parents with ankylosing spondylitis have a 25 to 50 per cent chance of inheriting the antigen but probably only a 1 in 20 chance of developing the disease. Genetic counselling is therefore unnecessary, but many patients now know that the disease can be inherited and will need reassurance.

Management

The aims of management are: maintenance of spinal mobility; prevention and correction of spinal deformity; relief of pain and stiffness.

MAINTENANCE OF SPINAL MOBILITY

The importance of physiotherapy cannot be overstated. However, since the patient may require to perform exercises for many years or even the rest of his life, it is vital that he be properly taught a simple programme of exercises. Further, the purpose of spinal and chest mobilising exercises must be explained and the patient frequently encouraged by doctor and therapist. Exercises may also be required for peripheral joints. Heat and other physical therapies have little value. Immobilisation in bed or spinal supports must be avoided.

Patients who continue playing a wide range of sports may consider this sufficient exercise, but it must be stressed that most sports involve spinal flexion and such individuals still need to undertake spinal extension exercises. The most useful test for the patient to assess his progress is the ability to stand with his heels, buttocks, shoulders and occiput against the wall. Any deterioration in this ability is the sign to increase the level of exercise.

PREVENTION OF SPINAL DEFORMITY

A firm bed, the use of one pillow, and a daily period of prone lying are essential. (Prone lying also discourages the tendency to hip flexion in those with early hip disease.) Further, the posture adopted at work or in the home is vital. The patient must always be conscious of his spinal posture and adapt his life, chairs and work situations accordingly. The occupational therapist and physiotherapist can implement this advice.

CORRECTION OF SPINAL DEFORMITY

Although immobilisation in bed should generally be avoided, there are some cases which have already deteriorated into a position of typical spinal deformity which can be greatly improved by an aggressive treatment programme. This requires admission to hospital for about two weeks during which, in addition to routine anti-inflammatory drugs, the disease process is further suppressed with a reducing course of corticosteroids. The first five days are spent supine in bed, gradually reducing the height of the pillows supporting the head until finally no pillow is required. Deep breathing exercises are practised several times daily. Bed exercises to mobilise the spine and strengthen the back muscles are introduced and must be practised vigorously and frequently. In the remaining days the patient spends less time supine and starts exercises in the standing position. Correction of posture in standing and sitting should be practised. At the same time the patient can be introduced to the benefits of prone lying which will correct early flexion deformities at the hips.

Following discharge from hospital the patient must follow a programme of exercises and activities listed under the headings of maintenance and prevention of spinal mobility and deformity.

RELIEF OF PAIN AND STIFFNESS

One of the analgesic/anti-inflammatory drugs listed on p. 222 should be used. Phenylbutazone and indomethacin are popular and bedtime doses relieve morning stiffness. For severe cases corticosteroids may be required. A short course of these drugs or ACTH may reduce pain and stiffness and muscle spasm and result in considerable increase in movement which the well-instructed patient can then maintain.

Radiotherapy, once popular, has largely been discarded since it caused an increased incidence of leukaemia in later years. However, radiotherapy may still be employed in cases genuinely unresponsive to other treatment.

Surgery

Posterior spinal osteotomy for spinal deformity is possible, but is both difficult and dangerous. Peripheral joint involvement may be treated by synovectomy and total hip replacement may dramatically alter a patient's life. Patients with ankylosing spondylitis are among the youngest currently undergoing hip replacement. Although there is a higher incidence of heterotopic bone formation, sometimes leading to ankylosis, than in other diseases, the results are generally satisfactory.

Prognosis

The prognosis is good and should encourage proper management. In general the mental attitude of the spondylitic is excellent and this should encourage the therapist. Almost all patients can remain at work and over half continue with their original employment. Problems mostly occur in those patients with insidious, long-standing disease who already have deformity and immobility when first seen. Early and continuing treatment is important.

REITER'S DISEASE

Reiter's disease is characterised by urethritis, sero-negative arthritis and conjunctivitis in young men.

Clinical Features

Although the presence of urethritis and arthritis are essential for the diagnosis to be made, conjunctivitis is not, since it is found in only half the cases. Mouth and genital ulceration and a characteristic skin lesion – keratoderma blennorrhagica – each occur in 10 per cent of cases. In Great Britain and Western Europe the disease usually develops from non-specific urethritis which is transmitted sexually. However, in some cases and particularly in many tropical and developing countries and in time of war, a similar disease, reactive arthritis, follows various types of dysentery (see p. 83). The venereal type of the disease is uncommon in women. Approximately 1 per cent of men with non-specific urethritis will develop other features of Reiter's disease after 10 to 21 days. The annual recurrence rate is about 15 per cent and can be precipitated by trauma and intercurrent infection as well as urethritis and dysentery.

URETHRITIS

A serous, sterile urethral discharge may be accompanied by dysuria and haematuria. Inflammation in other parts of the genito-urinary system with cystitis, prostatitis, salpingitis, etc. is not uncommon. Penile ulceration is common and the ulcers may coalesce to form the typical circinate balanitis in about 10 per cent of cases.

ARTHRITIS

This is an acute, asymmetrical arthritis negative for rheumatoid factor and involving mostly knees, ankles and feet, although any peripheral joint may be affected. There is marked synovial proliferation and effusion and often serious disability. Tendinitis and fasciitis, particularly around the ankle and heel, is common (Plate 7/4). With persistent or recurrent disease sacro-iliac joint involvement occurs and may progress to a patchy spondylitis making the differentiation from ankylosing spondylitis difficult. An erosive arthritis similar to rheumatoid arthritis occurs in some cases and may lead to serious deformity, particularly of the feet.

EYES

Conjunctivitis with sterile eye discharge causing overnight 'gumming'

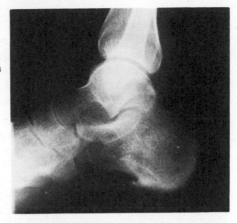

Plate 7/4 Radiograph showing plantar fasciitis in Reiter's disease. Note the large plantar spurs which appear fluffy due to the periosteal reaction

of the eyelids is the usual ocular sign. Iritis, with the danger of permanent eye damage, occurs in persistent and recurrent cases, usually those with sacro-iliac joint involvement.

SKIN AND MOUTH LESIONS

Non-specific mouth ulceration is common but a more characteristic ulcerated area may be found on the roof of the mouth in 10 per cent of cases.

Keratoderma blennorrhagica develops on the palms and soles in 10 per cent of cases. The deep-seated sterile pustules resemble those of pustular psoriasis. The involved skin becomes much thickened and there are accompanying destructive lesions of the nails.

OTHER FEATURES

A systemic reaction with fever, weight loss and general malaise is usual. Heart, lung and neurological involvement have been recorded but death from Reiter's disease is extremely rare.

RADIOLOGY

Early radiographs may show evidence of periostitis due to joint and tendon involvement, but later the appearances are difficult to distinguish from rheumatoid arthritis and ankylosing spondylitis, depending upon whether peripheral or spinal joints are involved.

Diagnosis and Aetiology

Blood tests show no characteristic features. The white cell count and ESR are raised and there is often a mild anaemia. Synovial fluid examination confirms the inflammatory nature of the disease but occasionally may show the presence of large macrophages, 'Reiter's cells'. All tests for infection are negative.

The important diseases to exclude are other venereal diseases, syphilis and gonorrhoea, which may produce urethritis and arthritis and which may co-exist with Reiter's disease. In later cases and especially in women, in whom the urethritis may be symptomless, the differentiation from ankylosing spondylitis and other causes of sacro-iliac joint inflammation is difficult. The skin lesions may be confused with those of psoriasis.

The cause is unknown although an infection seems likely. All attempts to reliably isolate an organism have failed. Undoubtedly genetic factors determine which patients with non-specific urethritis will proceed to Reiter's disease. Once again, there is an increased incidence of the tissue antigen HLA B27. The percentage of patients with positive tests is approximately 65 per cent in those with peripheral joint involvement rising to over 90 per cent in those who develop sacro-iliac and spinal disease (see p. 77). A patient with non-specific urethritis and a positive test has about a 1 in 15 chance of developing Reiter's disease.

Management

Management will include: 1) rest and splintage, 2) anti-inflammatory drugs, 3) joint aspiration and injection, 4) antibiotics and 5) surgery.

The disease is self-limiting in almost every case, but the time to remission varies from three weeks to two years. The aims of management are to induce early remission and certainly prompt treatment shortens the course of the disease. Full bed rest, usually with splints, is the quickest and ultimately the kindest way to settle the arthritis in impatient young men. Aspiration of joint effusion and intra-articular corticosteroids will speed this process. It is vital that mobilisation proceeds slowly as recurrence is common, especially if too much activity is allowed before muscle bulk has returned. The decision to mobilise must be taken clinically as the ESR is slow to settle and is a poor guide to management. Full dosage of an anti-inflammatory drug (p. 223) should be given and in cases failing to improve corticosteroids or even immunosuppressive agents may be required. Antibiotics, ideally oxy-tetracycline, will control the non-specific urethritis but will have no effect upon the rest of the disease.

In persistent or recurrent cases synovectomy or even reconstructive surgery, particularly of the feet, may be undertaken.

REACTIVE ARTHRITIS

Although it has been recognised that Reiter's disease may develop from dysenteric infections and that such infections may occasionally cause a septic arthritis, it has only recently been appreciated that more obvious non-suppurative arthritis, unassociated with the other features of Reiter's disease may follow often very mild dysentery, due to Shigella, Salmonella and Yersinia infections. As in Reiter's disease the arthritis, usually affecting the knees and ankles, produces a florid synovial response with a considerable systemic reaction of malaise, fever, raised white cell count and ESR. Although a short, self-limiting course is usual, occasional cases proceed to sacro-iliitis and patchy spondylitis.

The sex incidence is equal and over 90 per cent of patients carry the HLA B27 antigen. The diagnosis is often difficult since the patients may have forgotten or been unaware of the bowel infection which precedes the arthritis by 10 to 14 days. Stool culture and/or serological tests are positive for the organisms.

Treatment is the same as for Reiter's disease. Antibiotics have no effect and are only indicated when there is a continuing bowel infection.

PSORIATIC ARTHROPATHY

Psoriasis and rheumatoid arthritis are both common conditions each affecting 2 per cent of the population and may occur coincidentally in the same patient. However, a specific form of sero-negative polyarthritis is now recognised, and although the management is essentially the same as that of rheumatoid arthritis, the disease is associated with less systemic upset and has a better prognosis.

Clinical Features

The presence of psoriasis is essential for the diagnosis. However, only small patches on the extensor surfaces of knees and elbows or in the scalp may be found. Nail involvement, with pitting, ridging and/or destructive lesions, is very common. Occasionally in patients with a family history of psoriasis, the diagnosis may be suspected before the development of skin or scalp lesions and indeed with some patients there may be a delay of many years before the skin lesions appear. In the majority of cases, however, skin changes have been present for some years before arthritis develops. Four patterns of joint involvement are recognised although two or more patterns may co-exist.

DISTAL INTERPHALANGEAL JOINT DISEASE

This erosive arthritis of the hands and feet is often associated with marked bone loss of the finger tufts (Plate 7/5). Involvement of these joints is rare in rheumatoid arthritis but the features may be confused with generalised osteoarthrosis with Heberden node formation if nails and skin are not carefully examined.

RHEUMATOID TYPE DISEASE

The pattern of joint involvement follows that of rheumatoid arthritis although tending to be less symmetrical and more patchy and often accompanied by marked flexor tendon involvement producing a 'sausage' finger. The tests for rheumatoid factor remain negative.

SACRO-ILIAC JOINT DISEASE

Bilateral sacro-iliitis alone or in association with other patterns of disease is common, and may progress to spondylitis indistinguishable from ankylosing spondylitis.

ARTHRITIS MUTILANS

This is a rare, very destructive arthritis associated with marked bone loss which produces the appearance of telescoping of the soft tissues since their length is unaltered (Plate 7/6).

There are clear genetic influences in the disease since there is an increased incidence of psoriasis, psoriatic arthropathy and ankylosing

Plate 7/5 (*below*) Psoriatic arthritis of the hand showing nail and distal interphalangeal joint involvement

Plate 7/6 (*right*) Radiograph of a foot with psoriatic arthritis showing erosions of the distal interphalangeal joints of the foot with marked bone loss in the second toe

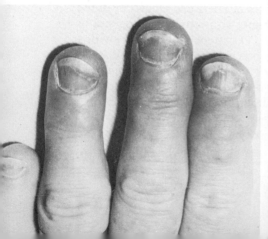

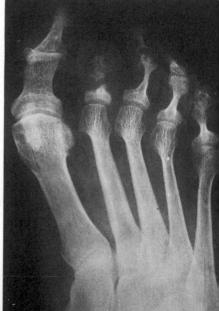

spondylitis in the patients' relatives. There are probably links with Reiter's disease and the arthropathy of ulcerative bowel disease.

Management

Exacerbations in the skin and joint disease rarely coincide and each must be treated separately. Skin lesions should be treated initially with a descaling ointment and various tar-based preparations are suitable. Subsequently local corticosteroid therapy is employed. Scalp lesions should be treated with a steroid lotion. The psoriasis may be sufficiently severe to seek the advice of a dermatologist. Unfortunately, successful treatment of the skin lesions has no effect upon the joint symptoms unless oral corticosteroids have been used. Treatment of the joints should follow the lines suggested for rheumatoid arthritis and ankylosing spondylitis. In most cases the benign nature of the disease means that an anti-inflammatory drug is all that is required, but more severe cases may require corticosteroids or even an antimetabolite such as methotrexate. The therapist can help with exercise programmes, local therapy to finger joints and general advice. Surgical procedures of the type used in rheumatoid arthritis may occasionally be required and are associated with similar results. Active skin lesions are no bar to surgery but extra preparation of these infected areas is advisable.

ULCERATIVE COLITIS AND CROHN'S DISEASE

These distinguishable diseases which present with severe diarrhoea and general ill-health are associated with similar articular features. These include:

COLITIC ARTHRITIS

This is a self-limiting synovitis and effusion, usually of the knees and ankles. A simple programme of rest, splints, anti-inflammatory drugs and exercises will control symptoms and restore full function. The arthritis mirrors the activity of the bowel disease and remits completely after colectomy.

SACRO-ILIITIS

Twenty per cent of patients have sacro-iliitis, leading to an increased incidence of ankylosing spondylitis. Iritis is a common complication. The usual management of ankylosing spondylitis is applicable.

ERYTHEMA NODOSUM

Ulcerative bowel disease may be associated with erythema nodosum (see p. 90).

BIBLIOGRAPHY

See end of Chapter 12.

Chapter 8

Inflammatory Arthritis

by A. G. MOWAT, M.B., F.R.C.P. (Ed.) and J. M. ABERY, M.C.S.P.

ARTHRITIS DUE TO INFECTIONS

Rheumatic Fever

Rheumatic fever is a disease of declining incidence and severity which affects young people and which is caused by an abnormal immunological reaction to infection with β-haemolytic streptococcus. The streptococcal infection is usually in the throat and although this may have cleared by the time other features of the disease appear, a rising anti-streptolysin (ASO) titre in the blood can be taken as evidence of infection. The most serious effect of rheumatic fever follows inflammatory damage to heart structures, often leading to mitral and aortic valve disease and cardiac arrhythmias, which will produce increasing disability during the rest of the patient's life, especially during episodes of cardiac strain such as pregnancy.

The acute stage of the disease is characterised by fever, polyarthritis, subcutaneous nodules, skin rash, chorea and a raised ESR. The polyarthritis migrates through any peripheral joint, accompanied for two to three days by marked swelling and pain but causing no permanent damage.

MANAGEMENT

Rest is essential for both the heart and joints in the acute phase of the disease. Splintage of joints is rarely necessary. Aspirin and related drugs (p. 223) dramatically relieve joint symptoms and control the fever. Corticosteroids are occasionally required for severe cases. Penicillin will eradicate any residual streptococcal infection and is generally given for five years to protect the patient against recurrent infection and subsequent rheumatic fever.

For the patient who has sustained cardiac damage, prophylactic antibiotic therapy may be required during any infective episode and particularly if teeth are to be extracted. In later life, these patients may require treatment for atrial fibrillation and cardiac failure, while a few may undergo mitral and aortic valve surgery.

Septic Arthritis

Septic arthritis may result from infection elsewhere in the body and from the introduction of bacteria directly into the joint by trauma, intra-articular injection or operation. Occasionally it may occur without obvious cause in a damaged joint. The presence of a metal prosthesis appears to increase the risk of such infection, and any debilitating disease, diabetes or treatment with corticosteroids and immunosuppressive agents, will further exaggerate the tendency to joint infection.

The patient is usually unwell, with fever, rigors and raised white cell count. The larger peripheral joints are usually affected but no joint is immune. Although the staphylococcus is the commonest infecting organism, infection with other organisms such as salmonella and meningococcus must be remembered.

MANAGEMENT

Prompt bacteriological culture of the synovial fluid, blood and any other potentially infected material is essential. Systemic treatment with the appropriate antibiotic and local support for the painful joint is given. Surgical drainage or irrigation of joints is seldom necessary. Repeated aspiration of a large effusion will make the patient more comfortable but local injection of antibiotic is unnecessary and may cause chemical irritation.

Gonococcal Arthritis

Gonorrhoea, an increasingly common venereal disease, may cause articular disease. The arthritis is commoner in women, particularly negresses, in whom the initial urethritis and other genito-urinary symptoms are often mild and untreated. The arthritis, most commonly in the knee, is a form of septic arthritis but is often preceded by a flitting arthralgia and accompanied by tenosynovitis and a rash. Diagnosis is more certain if it is suggested to the bacteriologist, as culture of the organism may be difficult. Antibiotic therapy should ensure a full remission.

Brucellosis

Despite testing of cattle, brucellosis may result from drinking unpasteurised milk. Direct contact with infected animals as a source of infection only applies to farmworkers, butchers and veterinary surgeons. There is intermittent fever, general malaise, myalgia and arthralgia of larger limb joints. A destructive, septic arthritis of hip, knee and spine may follow. Diagnosis is by serum agglutination test and treatment with streptomycin and tetracycline.

Tuberculosis

This is now a rare cause of arthritis, although the joint remains second to the lung as a site of infection. The disease is commoner and painful in children, but chronic, often relatively painless, monarticular disease should suggest tuberculosis in any age group, particularly in the elderly and in coloured immigrants. The hip, knee and lumbar spine are the usual sites of infection and involvement of tendons and fingers and the tracking of a 'cold' psoas abscess to the groin are now all rare. Diagnosis may be delayed, often being made after biopsy of involved areas. Treatment is with standard anti-tuberculous drugs and immobilisation. The patient should be referred to a chest physician, so that the patient and his contacts can be examined regularly for possible pulmonary tuberculosis, and given appropriate treatment. Without such referral, and the exclusion of tuberculous cows from milk production for public consumption, these two main forms of tuberculosis could again become widespread in the United Kingdom. Synovectomy of peripheral joints is indicated both for diagnostic and therapeutic reasons. Other surgical treatment is rarely needed in Britain.

Viral Arthritis

With increasingly sophisticated viral culture methods and reliable serological methods of measuring antibody levels, it has been appreciated that a transient, but often painful, synovitis may accompany many viral infections. Rubella (German measles) arthritis is the commonest, tending to affect the knees of young women, the group already at risk from this infection since it may cause fetal abnormalities. Arthritis may accompany influenza, mumps and measles in young adults but fortunately children are rarely affected. Transient arthritis, particularly of the fingers, may precede other signs of hepatitis associated with the Australia antigen and occasionally in such patients a life-threatening vasculitis resembling polyarteritis nodosa may develop. The diagnosis is often made after the symptoms have settled by finding a rise in the level of antibodies in the blood.

Erythema Nodosum

Erythema nodosum is characterised by crops of large, red, tender, raised lesions over the shins, which gradually fade like bruises. The rash represents a hypersensitivity reaction to a variety of causes including sarcoid, tuberculosis, streptococcal infection, ulcerative colitis, Crohn's disease and drug allergy. However, in up to one half of cases no cause is found. A synovitis, usually of the knees and ankles, occurs in some 60 to 70 per cent of patients with erythema nodosum. Confusion may arise since the synovitis often precedes the skin rash by several weeks. The synovitis settles over weeks or months even, without treatment, but salicylates or even corticosteroids should usually be given. Although the synovitis settles over a period of 3 to 12 weeks without treatment, simple anti-inflammatory drugs or corticosteroids should be given. Some patients require a long period of supervised rest with splintage.

CONNECTIVE TISSUE DISEASES

Disseminated Lupus Erythematosus

This disease, which is most common in young women, is associated with a characteristic facial rash, loss of scalp hair and synovitis of small, peripheral joints. These features represent the mildest form of the disease which with greater clinical awareness and the development of more sophisticated laboratory tests is being increasingly recognised. The joints may resemble those of early rheumatoid arthritis although cartilage and bone damage, and hence serious deformity and disability, are unusual.

However, many patients develop a wide range of serious lesions in internal organs and although severe disease tends to declare itself early, no patient, however long they have had the disease, can be considered immune from such complications. Several types of serious and often fatal renal disease frequently occur, while up to half the patients show evidence of central nervous system involvement with personality changes, psychotic states and fits. Myositis and pleurisy are common and due to the inflammatory damage in blood vessels almost any organ or tissue may be affected.

Anaemia and a raised ESR are common. Low white cell and platelet counts are common features of the disease and may result in inter-current infections or purpuric or haemorrhagic episodes. Proteinuria is the sign of renal involvement, and renal biopsy may be required to determine the type and severity of this involvement. Although a variety of abnormal antibodies have been found in this disease the significance of many is ill-understood. The finding of high levels of anti-DNA (deoxyribonucleic acid) and anti-nuclear antibodies in the serum and altered white cells, so called LE cells, in the peripheral blood, are the most useful diagnostic tests.

The disease carries a very variable prognosis depending upon the extent of the internal organ involvement particularly the kidney and central nervous system. Mild disease may be treated with anti-inflammatory drugs (p. 223) and chloroquine. Severe disease is usually treated with high doses of corticosteroids and immunosuppressive agents although there remains some doubt whether the latter very toxic drugs, really alter the natural history of the disease.

Dermatomyositis

This is a rare disease characterised by chronic, inflammatory disease in muscles, especially the proximal limb muscles. The patient complains of muscle tenderness and progressive weakness, and the serum levels of muscle enzymes (aldolase, creatine phosphokinase) are raised. Heliotrope (bluish purple) discolouration of the face and extensor surfaces of the fingers is found in dermatomyositis but is absent from the otherwise identical polymyositis. Both diseases show evidence of widespread vascular abnormalities including synovitis of peripheral joints but motility disturbance and other gastro-intestinal symptoms are the commonest. The disease is commoner in women and there are peak incidences in childhood and again in the fourth and sixth decades. The incidence of underlying neoplastic disease increases with the age of onset of the disease, and a careful hunt for a tumour should be made.

The prognosis is poor in children with only half surviving two years. Adults without tumour do better. High doses of corticosteroids are usually required.

Scleroderma (Progressive Systemic Sclerosis)

This is a rare disease which affects skin, joints, gastro-intestinal tract, lungs and kidneys. The disease may be confined to the skin for many years producing a tight, shiny appearance in hands and face. Skin atrophy and calcification may lead to ulceration and gangrene. Joint deformities may be produced. Synovitis in joints is usually mild.

The disease is often preceded by Raynaud's phenomenon – a hypersensitivity to cold demonstrated by whiteness and 'deadness' of the fingers. Raynaud's phenomenon is common in children but late onset or increasing severity of the phenomenon should suggest scleroderma or other connective tissue disease.

The prognosis in scleroderma is related to the age of onset and the severity of anaemia, renal and lung symptoms. At present there is no effective treatment for patients who have involvement of internal organs but the skin changes may be improved by D-penicillamine (p. 228).

Sjögren's Syndrome

This is a chronic inflammation of the lacrimal and salivary glands leading to dryness of the eye and mouth. In some two-thirds of cases rheumatoid arthritis or another connective tissue disease is present. Rarely there may be involvement of other glandular structures leading to reduced sweating, reduced bronchial and nasal secretions, reduced gastric and pancreatic secretions and vaginitis. The underlying connective tissue disease should be treated in the usual ways. There is no effective treatment for Sjögren's syndrome although corticosteroids may be tried. Eye damage can be prevented by using methyl cellulose drops ('artificial tears').

Polyarteritis Nodosa

The features of polyarteritis nodosa are due to patchy, inflammatory damage in medium-sized arteries. They include haematuria, hypertension and renal failure, myocardial infarction and arteritis, gastrointestinal haemorrhage and perforation, skin nodules, hemiplegia and peripheral neuropathy and polyarthritis. Larger joints are usually involved, synovitis being migratory and rarely leading to erosive or permanent changes. The disease differs from the other connective tissue diseases in affecting more men than women and in involving rather larger arteries. A proportion of patients have asthma and lung infiltration on chest radiographs. Such patients usually have a raised eosinophil count in the blood. Otherwise investigations, apart from biopsy of the lesions, are not helpful. The disease causes early death and there is no definitive treatment.

Polymyalgia Rheumatica

Polymyalgia rheumatica is a clinical syndrome of unknown cause in which severe pain, stiffness and tenderness of the muscles of the shoulder and pelvic girdles are accompanied by a variety of systemic symptoms and signs. These include general malaise, fever, loss of weight and appetite, headache and depression. The onset is frequently sudden, producing severe disability. Joint involvement is minimal. The ESR is markedly elevated but there are no other specific laboratory findings. There is no evidence of muscle disease.

An underlying vasculitis can be found by temporal or other artery biopsy in 25 per cent of cases and is probably the basis for the disease in all cases. Temporal (or giant cell) arteritis is a variant of the same disease. Corticosteroid therapy rapidly controls the muscular and generalised symptoms, and prevents the development of serious vascular symptoms (which include blindness). The disease, which occurs often in patients over 60 years, is self-limiting and treatment can be reduced and generally stopped after two or three years.

CRYSTAL ARTHRITIS

Gout

Gout represents the inflammatory response of some patients, usually men, to a raised plasma uric acid level (hyperuricaemia) and to the deposition in tissues of monosodium urate crystals.

CLINICAL FEATURES

Gout occurs in males, usually after the age of thirty, and is rare in women until the menopause. Studies of the beneficial effect of oestrogens on blood levels of uric acid and on the susceptibility of cells to damage by urate crystals explain this finding, but do not offer a satisfactory form of treatment.

The disease presents as an acute attack of crystal synovitis which clears completely in a week or so, to be followed at intervals of weeks, months or even years by further attacks. After a time deposits of urate, tophi, appear on the ears, in tendons and in joints. The joint disease becomes more chronic and leads to secondary degenerative joint disease. The acute attack, which frequently involves the metatarsophalangeal joint of the great toe, causes severe pain, redness, and swelling. There is usually a systemic reaction with malaise, fever and a raised ESR and white cell count. Any joint, including the spine, may be involved but it is uncommon in the hip and shoulder. Two per cent

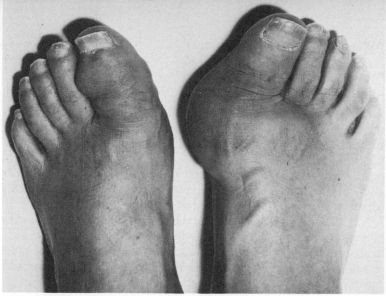

Plate 8/1 Gout. Note the typical swelling of the right first metatarsophalangeal joint and the tophaceous deposits in the left great toe

of cases are chronic from the outset. The incidence of tophi increases with the length of the history of gout and in untreated cases may reach 90 per cent (Plate 8/1). Tophi are only occasionally visible on radiographs. They may involve many organs and although they are present in 10 per cent of kidneys, the major renal abnormalities of fibrosis and vascular damage leading to hypertension and renal failure are caused by ill-understood mechanisms. Renal disease is a major cause of death in patients with gout.

METABOLIC AND PATHOLOGICAL MECHANISMS

Uric acid is the final breakdown product of purines and is excreted chiefly by the kidney. There are three major factors in purine metabolism: 1) the replacement and breakdown of body purines (endogenous); 2) the breakdown of ingested purines (dietary) and 3) the renal excretion of uric acid.

The plasma uric acid level and the incidence of gout depends upon the interaction of these factors. The upper limits of normal are usually taken as 0·40mmol/l for women and 0·50mmol/l for men. Approximately 5 per cent of the population has higher values and is thus hyperuricaemic but only a small proportion will develop gout.

THE REPLACEMENT AND BREAKDOWN OF BODY PURINES

The major pathways in purine metabolism are shown in Fig. 8/1. The amount of uric acid resulting from the breakdown of body purines is at least partly controlled by the ability of enzymes to salvage various purine metabolites (dotted lines in figure). The absence or reduced activity of such enzymes will result in increased uric acid production. Such enzyme abnormalities are probably genetically determined. The last stages in purine breakdown from hypoxanthine to xanthine to uric acid are controlled by the enzyme xanthine oxidase. This fact is utilised in the management of gout with the xanthine oxidase inhibitor allopurinol. Hyperuricaemia with attacks of gout is due to the overloading of this delicately balanced system by an increase in endogenous purine metabolism following a variety of stresses such as infection, surgery and trauma. Secondary gout is caused by excessive purine breakdown in the presence of a normal metabolic pathway and occurs in such diseases as the leukaemias, polycythaemia, myeloma and psoriasis.

BREAKDOWN OF INGESTED PURINES

This is not an important cause of gout as it is exceptional for patients to produce hyperuricaemia with even severe dietary excess unless there is some metabolic abnormality, of the type suggested above, already present. Dietary restriction is thus not necessary with current drug therapy.

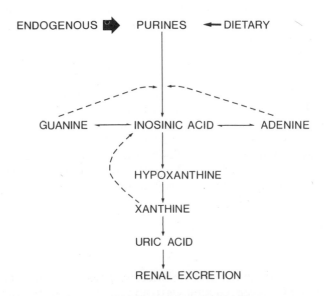

Fig. 8/1 The major pathways in purine metabolism

RENAL EXCRETION OF URIC ACID

The rate of excretion of uric acid is genetically determined and is proportional to the plasma uric acid levels. The excretion rate increases as the plasma level rises but in some patients the excretion rate is set at a lower level and hyperuricaemia and gout result. Clearly, renal disease of many types can interfere with the excretion of uric acid and can consequently cause gout. Possibly more important, a variety of drugs and other factors can impair the ability of a normal kidney to excrete uric acid. These include diuretics, salicylates in low doses and ketosis due to starvation, diabetes or excessive alcohol intake. Moderation of alcohol intake is thus sensible in the management of gout. Other drugs, such as aspirin in high doses and uricosuric drugs such as probenecid, increase the excretion of uric acid and are used in treatment.

PATHOLOGY

The attack of gout is caused by the ingestion of micro-crystals of urate by white cells in the synovial fluid with a subsequent release of inflammatory enzymes. Such attacks occur either when the solubility of urate in body fluids has been exceeded and deposits are accumulating, particularly in articular and periarticular tissues, or when the plasma uric acid is lowered and such deposits are going into solution. The second mechanism explains why attacks of gout may occur during the first weeks of treatment.

DIAGNOSIS

The commonest diagnostic confusion is with septic arthritis since both diseases produce severe pain, marked local inflammation and a raised white cell count. The finding of an elevated plasma uric acid level indicates hyperuricaemia and hence the possibility of gout. The diagnosis is confirmed by the clinical features and the finding of uric acid crystals in a joint effusion. Large, 'punched-out', juxta-articular, bony lesions on the radiograph are helpful but not diagnostic features (Plate 8/2).

Treatment of Gout

The patient must understand the basic abnormalities in gout if he is to be persuaded to accept continuous treatment. Such treatment consists of: 1) relief of the acute attack and 2) prevention of further attacks.

RELIEF OF ACUTE ATTACK

Colchicine, although effective, produces diarrhoea in full dosage and is now rarely used. Phenylbutazone (800mg per day) and indomethacin (200mg per day) are very effective and the dose can be progressively reduced over one week. Systemic or intra-articular steroids are rarely required.

PREVENTION OF FURTHER ATTACKS

This follows the reduction in the plasma uric acid and can be achieved either with uricosuric drugs (probenecid 1–2g per day), which increase the renal clearance of urate or by a xanthine oxidase inhibitor (allopurinol 300mg per day). The use of the latter drug allows purine metabolites to be excreted as xanthines (Fig. 8/1) rather than uric acid, and since xanthines are excreted much better than uric acid, the drug has advantages in patients with severe gout or renal disease. Because of the risk of precipitating acute attacks it is usual to add a small dose of phenylbutazone or indomethacin for the first three months of treatment.

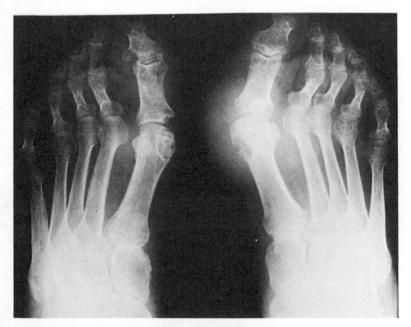

Plate 8/2 Radiograph of feet with gout (Plate 8/1), showing the soft tissue swelling and the bone erosions associated with deposits of uric acid

Pyrophosphate Arthropathy

This disease has a number of clinical expressions. The original description and the one most easily recognised, is of acute arthritis in the knees, wrists and shoulders of elderly patients which mimics acute gout and which has been called pseudo-gout. A single joint is usually involved and the diagnosis is made by finding typical calcium pyrophosphate dihydrate crystals in the synovial fluid. Characteristic radiological features are usually found in several joints, particularly the knee, shoulder, wrists and pubic symphysis, as well as the involved joint. These include calcification in both fibro and hyaline cartilage, but the presence of such calcification does not automatically make the diagnosis of pseudo-gout since many elderly patients show such features (Plate 8/3). The term chondrocalcinosis is best used to describe the radiographic features and not the disease. The disease is occasionally associated with hyperparathyroidism and haemochromatosis. Although the causative mechanism in this crystal

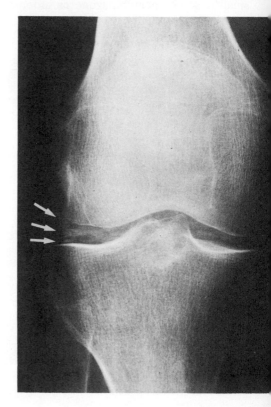

Plate 8/3 Radiograph of right knee with pyrophosphate arthropathy

arthritis is similar to that in gout, its response to anti-inflammatory drugs is less predictable and several such drugs may need to be tried before the best agent is found. The most effective treatment is joint aspiration and instillation of steroid. Long term treatment may be required to prevent further attacks.

It has become clear that reactive damage due to the presence of pyrophosphate crystals in the synovial fluid and tissue may produce other patterns of joint disease than acute synovitis. These include:

1. A widespread, sub-acute polyarthritis, often involving finger joints which imitates rheumatoid arthritis.
2. A neuropathic arthritis usually of the ankle joints.
3. Osteoarthrosis usually in the hip. This finding has challenged the view that osteoarthrosis is simply due to 'wear and tear', and has led to the re-introduction of the term 'osteoarthritis'.

In these variants the identification of typical crystals in synovial fluid or tissue may be very difficult while typical calcific radiographic features may be minimal and easily overlooked.

ARTHRITIS ASSOCIATED WITH MALIGNANT DISEASE

A variety of vague musculo-skeletal pains may be associated with any malignant disease, and bone pain from skeletal metastases is most common with lung, breast, thyroid and prostatic tumours. Leukaemia often presents with migratory polyarthritis and in children may be confused with rheumatic fever and juvenile chronic polyarthritis. Myeloma may present with polyarthritis either by direct involvement or by causing the deposition of amyloid tissue in and around joints.

Hypertrophic pulmonary osteoarthropathy, characterised by chronic periostitis of the distal limb bones at the wrists and ankles, recurrent synovitis of large joints and clubbing of the fingers is usually associated with lung and gastric tumours. Other associated conditions include liver cirrhosis, lung sepsis, and bacterial endocarditis. The pathological mechanisms involved are not clearly understood.

Despite the capacity of synovial tissue to proliferate in response to many irritants, a synovial tumour is very rare.

ARTHRITIS ASSOCIATED WITH HAEMOPHILIA

The most crippling complication of haemophilia is arthritis. This disorder, due to a deficiency of a blood clotting factor (factor VIII or anti-haemophilic globulin, AHG) is genetically determined, being transmitted by women but appearing as a clinical condition in men. The disease is characterised by repeated episodes of bleeding into joints and muscles and occasional bleeding from the kidney and gastro-intestinal tract, occurring from childhood onwards and often without an obvious cause. Joint and muscle haemorrhage causes severe pain, swelling and disability and if treated poorly or if the haemorrhages are frequent, permanent deformity results.

Management

The aims of management are to 1) control the bleeding, 2) relieve pain and 3) maintain and restore function.

CONTROL OF BLEEDING

Factor VIII must be replaced in sufficient quantity to allow normal blood clotting to proceed. With minor bleeding fresh plasma will suffice but with major bleeding some concentrate of plasma must be used. Factor VIII from animal sources can be used until antibodies develop and then a concentrate of human plasma prepared by various freezing techniques is employed. It is usual to employ factor VIII to control the initial haemorrhage and also to 'cover' the patient during early mobilisation. In addition, considerable quantities of factor VIII are required for several days if reconstructive surgery is undertaken to improve the function in damaged joints. This is a developing field in orthopaedic surgery.

RELIEF OF PAIN

Routine analgesics are employed. Anti-inflammatory drugs such as aspirin and phenylbutazone should be avoided as they further alter blood clotting. Rest in plaster of Paris splints will relieve pain and assist in the control of bleeding and tissue swelling.

MAINTENANCE AND RESTORATION OF FUNCTION

A continuing programme of splints and slow, careful mobilisation with suitable exercises, particularly for the quadriceps muscles, will maintain and restore function and for those with more severely dam-aged joints fixation splints may be needed (see Chapter 9).

ARTHRITIS ASSOCIATED WITH NEUROLOGICAL DISEASE

Paralysis of a limb may protect joints from both rheumatoid arthritis and osteoarthritis. However, partial nerve damage may exaggerate osteoarthrosis, since unusual joint loading may occur. Damage to the neurological supply of a joint may lead to gross destruction and instability (Charcot joint). Although the joint usually becomes pain-less, contrary to popular belief, the recurrent episodes of swelling earlier in the disease are often painful. Syringomyelia is the usual cause of this type of arthritis in the upper limb, while syphilis (tabes dorsalis) and diabetes are common causes in the lower limb joints. Repeated intra-articular steroid injections may rarely be the cause.

Treatment can be difficult. Analgesic drugs are helpful in the early stages but later, the patients complain of instability and associated disability, particularly if a lower limb joint is involved. Suitable bracing may be required. Surgical treatment should be embarked upon with caution. Arthroplasty, even with total joint replacement, is usually unsuccessful as bone destruction continues; arthrodesis, the logical answer to a severely damaged joint, may be attended by a high rate of non-union and hence the need for continued external support.

BIBLIOGRAPHY

See end of Chapter 12.

Chapter 9

The Management of Inflammatory Joint Disease

by A. G. MOWAT, M.B., F.R.C.P. (Ed.) and J. M. ABERY, M.C.S.P.

GENERAL PRINCIPLES OF MANAGEMENT

The same general principles of management apply to all forms of inflammatory joint disease in which the precise cause is unknown. However, the extent to which these principles are applied will depend upon the natural history, severity and chronicity of the disease. It is convenient to describe the general management of rheumatoid arthritis, and such treatment can be modified to suit each individual patient and disease. Indeed, the importance of planning the management of each patient cannot be over-emphasised. Better results are achieved in many forms of joint disease, particularly rheumatoid arthritis, if the patient is admitted to hospital early in the course of the disease. This reflects how important it is that the nature of the disease and the aims of treatment be fully understood by the patient, his family and his medical advisers from the onset.

There are considerable advantages in treating patients with inflammatory joint disease in a separate ward or unit as they can often help and advise each other and are not subjected to the pressures of bed turnover which inevitably prevail in general medical or surgical wards. These patients progress slowly and indeed may not improve if their treatment programmes are hurried. Further, since the diseases produce complex disabilities and are usually associated with domestic, economic, employment and social factors, team work is essential in their management. The team is composed of general practitioner, physician, orthopaedic surgeon, physiotherapist, occupational therapist, nursing staff and medical social worker. A psychiatrist may often be added. A close liaison must be continued with the various domiciliary services.

The aim of management of chronic joint disease is simply to allow the patient to achieve and maintain the maximum functional capacity. This will entail not only an accurate assessment of the initial status of the patient but a continuing assessment of the changing status of the disease and of the patient's reaction to the disease. It is important to appreciate that the patient's problem is not arthritis but rather the disability that the arthritis produces. Thus many patients, especially the elderly, are subjected to unnecessary hospital visits for examination and treatment when all they require is a simple, common sense approach to their domestic difficulties. There are no general rules about management. Each patient must be treated as an individual.

Such management may include the use of:

1. rest
2. exercise and other physical methods including walking aids
3. splintage
4. drugs (see p. 222)
5. nursing care and dietary advice
6. various appliances designed to overcome or reduce disability and dependence upon others
7. the introduction of changes in employment and in the pattern of daily living
8. orthopaedic surgery (see p. 167).

Role of the Physiotherapist

The physiotherapist is an important member of the management team and she has a varied role. The therapist's initial role must be (i) the assessment of the patient as a whole, temperamentally, socially and psychologically and, in particular, to try and determine which patients are likely to be able to co-operate fully with the therapist; (ii) the assessment and recording of muscle strength and quality according to standard scales, particularly around the joints with the major involvement; (iii) the measurement and recording of the ranges of active and passive joint movement, once again concentrating upon the joints chiefly affected.

Clearly, normal working time and the concentration of both patient and therapist does not allow highly detailed measurements of all joints and muscles to be made. It is important that the therapist should have the ability to spot the problems and so limit her examination and measurements. Further, it is important that she be able to record her findings in a simple manner so that she contributes to the general discussion of a patient's needs during conferences of the management team. Some form of charting sequential information is valuable and can be included in the patient's records (see p. 182).

The physiotherapist can do much to help the patient settle into hospital by giving a simple explanation of the disease process and relating this to the patient and his own disability. She should also be at hand to discuss with the patient what the doctor has said and the treatment he has ordered. Patients are often afraid to question doctors about their treatment in case they appear to be questioning its desirability. They welcome the possibility of discussing it with someone else who has experience of the methods of treatment. Further, she must assist in the general assessment of the patient's attitude to his disease and disability. A general discussion of the patient's and family's roles, the degree of protection of the patient by the family and the extent of insight of the patient into his or her present and potential problems, can be undertaken at the same time as a detailed assessment of muscle quality and strength is made.

Rest

For the patient at home a period of rest each day may allow increased and more economical function during the remainder of the day. Such a rest may be combined with the use of a suitable splint together with periods of prone and supine lying to prevent and/or correct deformity in the spine, hips and knees. For the patient with very active disease rest in hospital is required. The continued use of joints during a phase of active disease increases pain, muscle spasm and wasting and exaggerates any systemic symptoms, and tends to cause flexion deformities in weight-bearing joints. Bed rest relieves these symptoms and improves the general well-being of the patient. There are dangers, however, in uncontrolled bed rest in the form of general physical deterioration, muscle weakness and joint contractures.

Accordingly, splints for arms and legs are provided. The use of a firm mattress and a back rest to ensure adequate support, proper posture and comfort are necessary. A fixed bed cage with padded foot rest to keep the weight of the bedclothes off inflamed joints, to prevent foot drop during periods when leg splints are not worn, and to prevent the patient from slipping down the bed, is also necessary. Many patients prefer a continental quilt.

EXERCISE AND OTHER PHYSICAL METHODS INCLUDING WALKING AIDS

Exercise

There is little benefit in instituting physical exercises until joint activity has settled as it is very difficult to increase muscle bulk or strength around an actively inflamed joint. However, once the joint inflammation has settled, a planned programme of graduated exercises is essential as considerable muscle wasting occurs in association with joint disease. Elaborate exercise programmes are not necessary and will certainly not be undertaken by patients at home. Passive movements tend to produce protective muscle spasm and are discouraged. Active, isotonic exercises against increasing resistance are the most satisfactory; but where pain is still present on joint movement, and particularly for the knee joint, the exercises are performed isometrically.

Thus for the patient with painful knees associated with synovial proliferation and effusion, the period of rest in splints can be used by the therapist to discuss general aspects of his disease. The exercise programme is begun slowly, often allowing the patient to simply loosen up for the first two to three days. The use of a slippery board is helpful. The first exercises will be quadriceps contractions performed isometrically. The patient should be encouraged to achieve a modest target which can be repeated frequently during the day. When ten contractions can be achieved without fatigue, straight leg raising and flexion exercises can be commenced. The patient slowly progresses to straight leg raising with 2 to 4lb weights (depending on body build) attached to the ankles before weight-bearing is allowed. The last few

Plate 9/1 A 'hump' to aid extension of the knee and to improve the strength of the quadriceps postoperatively

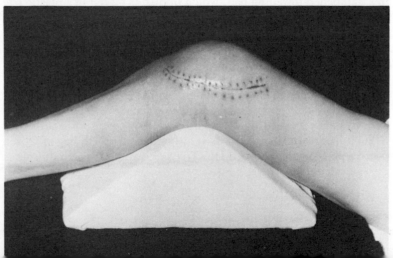

degrees of extension may be more readily achieved by supporting the knee over a small 'hump' (Plate 9/1). Weight-bearing initially involves standing by the bed and sitting down again, followed by marking time to allow the patient to regain balance and co-ordination. Early ambulation may require a walking aid.

Any increase in swelling, ache or pain, or any increase in morning stiffness, indicates that too much has been undertaken the previous day. Ice treatment will control these symptoms. The rate of increase in activity needs to be slower than many imagine.

Similar exercise programmes can be planned for any joint.

During any programme of rest and splintage for a joint or joints, general exercises designed to improve circulation and maintain muscular condition should be given to the remaining joints and trunk. The same considerations apply during the non-weight-bearing phase following orthopaedic surgical procedures.

Heating and Cooling

There are markedly different individual patient reactions and responses to heat and ice treatment and it is vital to select the correct treatment for each patient. Many inflamed joints are made worse by the application of heat but finger joints frequently respond to wax therapy. The therapist should assess each patient individually and be prepared to change from heat to ice and vice versa for the treatment of any joint.

Heat may be given by means of radiant heat, infra-red or short wave diathermy for large joints, while paraffin wax (melting point 38° to 41°C) is the best heat treatment for hands. Home treatment may be carried out by means of a hot water bottle enclosed in a blanket, a small electric heat pad for the hands or by the wearing of plastic gloves and holding the hands in a bowl of hot water.

However many patients prefer ice treatment. Chipped ice is placed in a dampened towelling bag, which in turn is placed in a plastic bag and put directly over the joint and left for 15 to 30 minutes. Ice treatment for the hands and wrists is best achieved by immersing them in melting ice for periods of up to 30 seconds until aching is produced. If this proves too painful, an ice bag, as for larger joints, can be used. Blanching of the fingers is an indication that they should be taken out and active exercise given immediately. In any event, ice treatment for the hands is best interspersed with exercises but for larger joints exercises are preceded by ice treatment.

Such ice treatment can be used at home using a 2lb bag of frozen peas in place of the chipped ice. The same application technique is used and after use the peas may be returned to the deep-freeze to be re-used many times.

Hydrotherapy is a form of treatment which produces widely differing results from different patients, and indeed there are marked differences among physiotherapists in their enthusiasm for an assessment of the value of such treatment. Unfortunately, there are no properly documented scientific studies of hydrotherapy and most comments are therefore personal in nature. These authors feel that hydrotherapy probably does not increase the final range of joint movement or reduce the time needed to achieve full weight-bearing, but it may improve a patient's morale.

Most patients enjoy exercise in the pool and are greatly encouraged by the movement they achieve in the water. The warmth and support of the water will reduce muscle spasm and pain and therefore increase the range of movement. Exercises can be given using the water to assist or resist movement. Functional activities such as sitting to standing, walking and step training are often easier to perform first in the water. More than one joint can be exercised in the water and this is of considerable value for patients with hip disease who also require mobilisation of the lumbar spine or knee. Over recent years, methods based on proprioceptive neuromuscular facilitation techniques have been in practice. By using appropriate floats the patient is completely buoyant. The physiotherapist positions her hands to facilitate the required movement and provides a fixed point around which the patient moves through the water. These techniques are found to be very valuable in the treatment of hip disease.

Faradism. After a period of bed rest many patients complain of pain under the feet, frequently at the site of insertion of the plantar fascia in the front of the heels. The authors have found that a short course of faradism given fairly strongly and combined with foot exercises is beneficial. It should be given by using wet pads and not by using a faradic foot bath.

Ultrasound may be useful in the treatment of a persistently painful ligament or joint capsule.

Crutches

Various forms of walking aids may be required and care must be taken in their selection. In many hospitals this is the responsibility of the physiotherapist. Many patients resist the idea of walking aids and a sympathetic explanation of the mechanics of weight relief may be needed.

The traditional axillary crutch is neither suitable nor necessary for most patients with joint disease. These crutches are designed largely or completely to relieve weight-bearing in one limb and impose considerable strain on upper limb joints and muscles, particularly the shoulder joint. A lightweight support which will provide some reduction in lower limb weight-bearing and increase confidence in walking is all that most patients require. Such supports may be used in one or both hands. The standard elbow crutch fills these needs (Fig. 9/1 A). However, the crutch cannot be used by patients with significant flexion deformity at the elbow, a painful wrist or very poor hand function. The alternative gutter crutch can be used by most of these patients since it demands even less of the upper arm joints; and, if fixed to the forearm by Velcro or other simple release fastening, can be managed even with severely affected hands (Fig. 9/1 B). The crutch height should always be adjustable and it is preferable to use crutches in which the length and position of the arm supports are also adjustable.

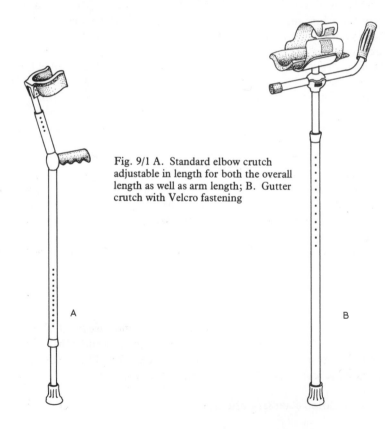

Fig. 9/1 A. Standard elbow crutch adjustable in length for both the overall length as well as arm length; B. Gutter crutch with Velcro fastening

A

B

Other Walking Aids

Walking sticks or a sturdy umbrella help many patients once they have overcome their pride. A single stick or crutch can be used by patients with unilateral disease to relieve weight and should be used on the contralateral side. However, better weight relief and balance are provided by the use of two supports. The sticks should be of the correct height; level with the greater trochanter with the patient erect in shoes or level with the lower end of the ulna with the arm held at the side. The handle of many sticks and crutches is too small for the arthritic hand to grip strongly, but soft padding, Sorbo-rubber or Plastazote can be used to provide the correct sized handle. Strong,

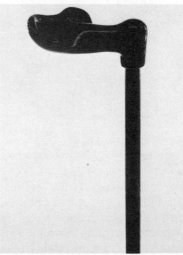

Plate 9/2 A right hand moulded walking stick handle

lightweight, inexpensive metal sticks with suitable, moulded left or right handles are available and these can be cut to the correct length (Plate 9/2). A straight handle is often preferred to the traditional curved handle. A very hard grip or a stick which is too long, causing wrist extension, may lead to symptoms of local median nerve compression.

Sticks with four small legs (quadruped) provide more support and are useful in those patients with poor balance whether due to neurological, eye or joint disease (Fig. 9/2 A). Most crutches and walking aids can be modified to provide a hook for a shopping basket or handbag. A lightweight, wide-based walking frame is favoured by many patients, particularly in the early stages of rehabilitation after surgery or severe disability. Occasionally patients with poor hand function cannot manage the walking frame, and a modified version

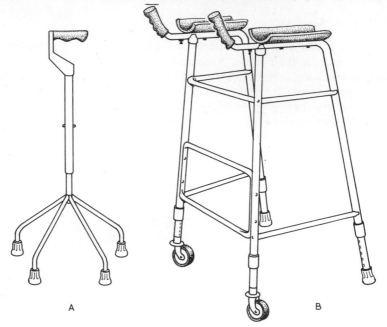

A   B

Fig. 9/2 A. A quadruped walking aid; B. A quadruped walking frame with
small wheels on leading legs, and arm supports

with two small wheels on the leading legs and suitably adjusted arm
supports should be provided (Fig. 9/2 B).

It must be emphasised that these frames should only be used in the
early stages of retraining in walking and that very few patients should
take them home from hospital. Undoubtedly some patients find the
wide open spaces of hospital wards and corridors disconcerting and
their confidence can be maintained by the use of a walking frame.
However, such aids do not encourage a normal walking movement
and since they are cumbersome in most small-roomed houses, the
patient should be converted to crutch or stick walking before discharge. Carefully positioned furniture will be found as useful in many
homes, but in other cases, a small trolley may be preferred since it
provides both a walking aid and a carrying surface. The patient may
need to be shown how to walk with a normal gait, climb stairs and rise
from a chair.

SPLINTAGE

Splints have three main functions: 1) rest and relief from pain,

2) prevention and correction of deformity and 3) fixation of a damaged joint in a good functional position.

Rest Splints

For the immediate treatment of a single, swollen and inflamed joint a vacuum splint provides adequate comfortable support. However, for those with several inflamed joints and for longer term use custom-made plaster of Paris splints are required. Skin-tight, unpadded plaster of Paris splints which hold the limb in good position without muscle spasm are bandaged on at night and for periods of rest during the day as long as active disease persists. Contrary to what might be expected, morning stiffness is decreased by the use of night splints as inflammation is controlled. The fear of joint stiffness progressing to ankylosis leads many to combine splinting with exercises, even during the most active phases of disease. However, there is no substance in these fears and as long as cartilage remains, joints do not become ankylosed.

Continuous immobilisation by fixing the splints to the limb with plaster cuffs, perhaps for three weeks, has a place in the early stages of rheumatoid arthritis (Fig. 9/3). It is probably best avoided in those

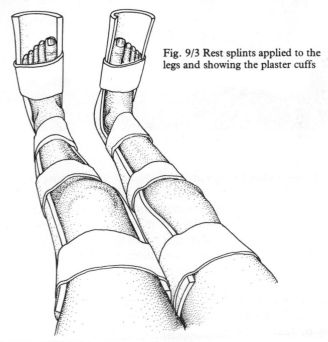

Fig. 9/3 Rest splints applied to the legs and showing the plaster cuffs

with severe joint damage and in elderly patients who more readily develop complications such as venous thrombosis, fluid retention, hypostatic pneumonia, constipation and osteoporosis. After removal of the rest splint from the limb, no formal exercises are performed for two to three days. However, gentle flexion is allowed and the use of a slippery board facilitates this in lower limb joints.

These splints are comfortable and allow no significant movement. They are made by direct application of plaster of Paris to a limb previously oiled with olive oil. Posterior shells extend from the gluteal creases to the heels with right-angled foot-plates and with knees in 3 to 5° of flexion. The patient lies prone with the leg supported on a

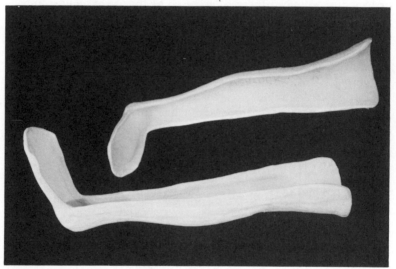

Plate 9/3 Plaster of Paris leg splints

sandbag. Some knee flexion must be allowed so that muscles relax and so that the foot can be held in mid-flexion without inversion. Posterior arm splints extend from the elbow to the finger tips with the wrist held in mid-pronation and a few degrees of extension. It is usual to leave one elbow free or the patient cannot reach her mouth. If the wrist and fingers are very deformed, anterior splints are easier to make and use. The minimum amount of plaster consistent with the patient's weight and strength is used. Care is taken in the finishing stages to remove all rough areas and the application of a fibreglass backing increases their strength and useful life (Plate 9/3). The making of splints is described fully on p. 123.

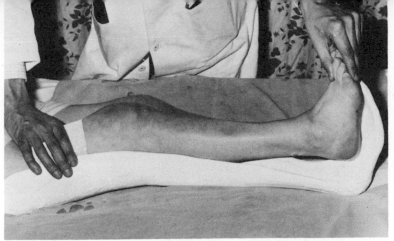

Plate 9/4 Plaster of Paris leg splints being used to correct a flexion deformity of the knee joint

Corrective Splints

Correction of deformity before contractures have occurred can be achieved at any joint, especially the knee, with the use of serial splints. The posterior shell, made as described above, is applied in the position of deformity, and no force, traction or manipulation is used. The shell is fixed to the limb with plaster cuffs. Symptoms settle rapidly and new splints which accommodate the gain in extension can be made at weekly intervals (Plate 9/4). When no further extension can be achieved, routine muscle strengthening exercises are used as a prelude to either walking or surgical treatment.

A similar correction may be achieved with dynamic reversed slinging, but it is important to ensure that excessive force is avoided lest joints be damaged or encouraged to sublux. Adequate analgesia and muscle relaxants must be given (Figs. 9/4 and 9/5).

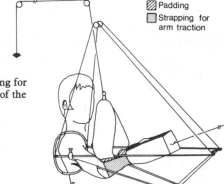

Fig. 9/4 Dynamic reversed slinging for correction of a flexion deformity of the elbow joint

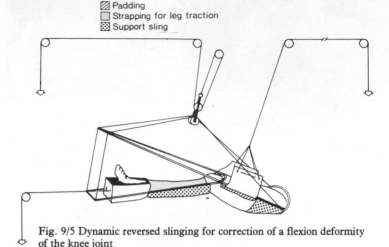

Fig. 9/5 Dynamic reversed slinging for correction of a flexion deformity of the knee joint

Walking and Working Splints

Static support for a persistently painful, unstable or permanently deformed joint can be provided by a removable splint. The splint is used to hold the joint in a position of function. Thus, to improve walking it may be necessary to use such splints on the knee or ankle and in addition splints can be used at the wrist and elbow joints, to improve the handling and value of suitable walking aids. Splints of this type allow the activity in a single joint or limb to settle without the need for complete rest. In addition, they can be used to reassure patients that any planned surgical fixation of a joint will not produce the disability that they fear. They are particularly useful long-term aids to function in patients who for various reasons may not be considered suitable for surgical treatment.

A variety of suitable materials exists such as Polythene, Orthoplast, leather and fibreglass, all of which combine lightness, strength and durability with ease of construction and use. Plastazote, although possessing some of these qualities, generally lacks the strength necessary for limb fixation; plaster of Paris is too heavy and many newer plastics are unnecessarily rigid and tend to cause local sweating. Velcro or similar simple fastenings should be used and care taken to ensure they are placed so that the patient can use them.

It is important that the splints should be fitted in the optimal position. Ideally an elbow should be held in 90° of flexion with the forearm in mid-pronation, and a wrist should be held in 10° of

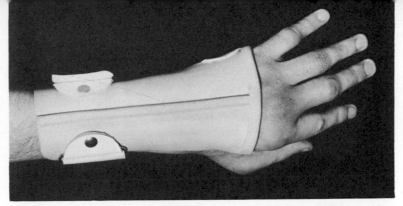

Plate 9/5 A light weight Prenyl working wrist splint with Velcro fastenings. A thin palmar band does not impair hand grip

extension with the thumb left free and finger flexion allowed, by using a dorsal splint with a thin palmar band (Plate 9/5). A knee is best supported by a full cylinder with the joint held in 5° of flexion and this can be removed for sitting (Fig. 9/6). Although, theoretically, the knee can be supported by a hinged caliper which allows the patient to sit easily, in practice it is often difficult to produce a cosmetically acceptable lightweight caliper and the multiple straps and hinge mechanism often cannot be managed by arthritic hands. Flexion deformities should be corrected as far as possible before supporting splints are provided for lower limb joints. Thus uncorrected knee deformities will tend to produce similar compensatory deformities at the hip and ankle joints in the same limb, and unless the inequality in leg length is corrected, similar deformities will develop in the opposite limb. Unfortunately many knee joints have a valgus deformity, and

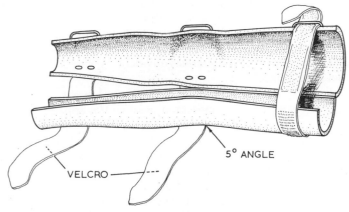

Fig. 9/6 Bi-valved fibre glass cylinder for support of the knee joint with Velcro fastenings

this makes the provision of a splint difficult since it will inevitably rub on the opposite knee.

Adequate fixation splints with simple fastenings are difficult to produce for the ankle joints. It is often simplest to provide a pair of boots or bootees. An alternative is to use a moulded posterior plastic splint stretching from mid-calf to mid-tarsus. This splint, which is fixed with a Velcro strap round the calf, also fixes the sub-talar joint (Fig. 9/7). Fixation of the sub-talar joint or correction of the common valgus deformity may also be achieved by the use of small plastic heel cups (Fig. 9/8), suitable insoles or firmly heeled shoes. An outside leg iron with or without a 'T' strap is very satisfactory but is not always cosmetically acceptable.

Broadening and rigidity of the forefoot with clawing of the toes and the developing of plantar callosities is particularly common in inflammatory joint disease, and can be helped by the use of metatarsal domed insoles. Great care must be taken to place the dome just proximal to the metatarsal heads, otherwise the insole will be ineffective or even increase foot pain. As these insoles take up space in shoes, new, larger shoes may be required if the insoles are to be used properly.

The greatest improvement in walking may be achieved by the provision of satisfactory shoes. In the early stages wider and deeper shoes with rigid soles and good supporting heel cups can be obtained from normal retail sources. With progressive disease it may be necessary to provide custom-made shoes. There has been some controversy over the advantages and disadvantages of seamless or 'space' shoes versus traditional surgical shoes. Seamless shoes are cheaper and tend to become available to the patient sooner but are unsightly to many wearers and tend to increase the sweating of the feet. Local arrangements often determine decisions; the speed of delivery, the accuracy of fitting and the ease of alteration are the key factors and these will vary from supplier to supplier. Patients with poor peripheral circulation, whether due to arteriosclerosis or vasculitis, should be provided with soft, fur-lined boots.

Finally every patient with lower limb joint or lower spinal involvement should have their legs measured. Real and/or apparent shortening of one leg is a common cause of symptoms in the contralateral, 'long' leg and in the lower back. The shoe should be raised approximately one-half the leg length difference in young patients and three-quarters of the difference in elderly patients. Such raises should not significantly increase the weight of the shoe. Raises of over 4 to 5cm (1½ to 2in) will need to be combined with sub-talar joint support, usually as a boot. With higher shoe raises some tapering of the sole allows the patient to walk more easily.

Fig. 9/7 (*right*) A moulded posterior
plastic splint for fixation of the ankle and
sub-talar joints

Fig. 9/8 (*below*) Moulded plastic heel cups
for either fixation of the sub-talar joint or
the correction of a common valgus
deformity

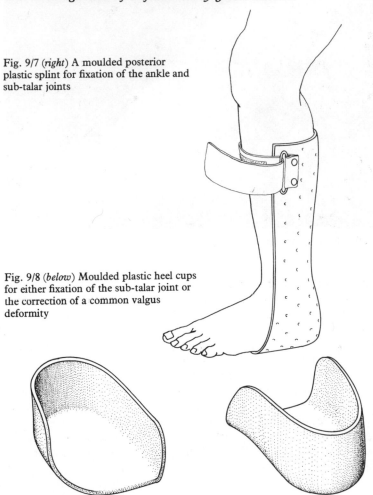

Protective Splint

Thinning of the skin particularly over the shins can be a problem in
patients with rheumatoid arthritis and this is discussed further in
Chapter 12. Although drug therapy, particularly corticosteroids and
penicillamine, may exaggerate this tendency it is essentially a feature
of the rheumatoid process and the amount of skin thinning is related
to the duration and severity of the disease. In addition there is a
reduction in the amount of supporting tissue to underlying blood
vessels so large bruises can develop with the slightest trauma.

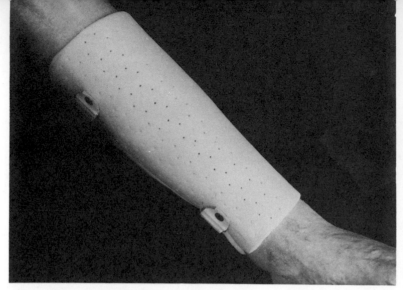

Plate 9/6 Plastazote shin guards

Further, tangential shearing stresses can easily remove a large area of skin leaving a lesion which is difficult to heal and which occasionally requires skin grafting.

Patients with such thin skin must be warned of the dangers of knocking into the furniture at home and particular care must be taken in hospital where there are metal beds and where they may easily be knocked in getting in and out of wheelchairs for transport to other departments. The wearing of slacks made of thicker material is often the only protection required and is currently an acceptable fashion for almost all patients. For those who are not prepared to adopt such a fashion or who have particularly thin and vulnerable skin the wearing of shin guards made of either Plastazote or leather is a satisfactory solution (Plate 9/6).

NURSING CARE AND DIETARY ADVICE

Nursing Care

The pain, stiffness, deformity and disability of joint disease make heavy demands on the nursing staff. The first few hours of each day can be difficult as this is the period of greatest disability for the patient. There is little value in demanding much of the patient in terms of washing, dressing, physical therapy, visits to X-ray, etc. until this period has passed. It is desirable that the beds should be of an adjustable height to facilitate the movement of patients and it is useful to have available hoists and other lifting devices. Toilets and bathrooms must be provided with adequate grab-rails, adjustable seats and non-slip mats. Many patients find showers simpler to use.

Patients who are immobilised in bed require regular turning; and if their limbs are fixed in splints, they may require assistance with feeding, washing, etc. Particular care must be paid to the condition of the skin or pressure sores will develop, particularly in those patients receiving steroid drugs and in those with systemic disease. The presence in the bed of small fragments of plaster of Paris is an added hazard. However, with proper nursing care, pressure sores should not develop and they certainly should not be accepted as an inevitable sequel to sustained bed rest in these patients.

Diet

Many patients suggest that an abnormal diet may have contributed to their development of rheumatoid arthritis or other joint disease. There is no evidence to support these suggestions. Patients require only a good balanced diet. It should be remembered that a number of patients are overweight and that this is an added burden to inflamed or damaged joints. A programme of weight reduction can usefully be instituted in hospital.

DOMESTIC AND OCCUPATIONAL FACTORS

Consideration of domestic and occupational factors produced by joint disease involves chiefly the occupational therapist and medical social worker, but satisfactory adaptation to disease depends upon the efforts of the whole medical team. In addition, these efforts are wasted unless the full co-operation of the patient and his family is obtained.

The traditional role of the occupational therapist has been to provide diversional activities during the patient's hospital stay. There remains a place for this in patients who may be in hospital for several weeks, but the activity should be chosen to ensure that it develops and improves functions in which the patient has become inefficient. The therapist should assess the patient's functional capacity in considerable detail as it is only in that way that sensible programmes of management can be arranged. It is helpful if there are facilities for the practice of routine activities such as dressing, bathing, cooking, ironing and the use of electrical equipment. Consideration can also be given to the provision of a wide range of gadgets to assist the patient with washing, dressing, eating, cooking, turning taps, etc. Ideally the patient should also be studied in his or her own home (Plate 9/7). Most of these gadgets and appliances are very simple and physiotherapists

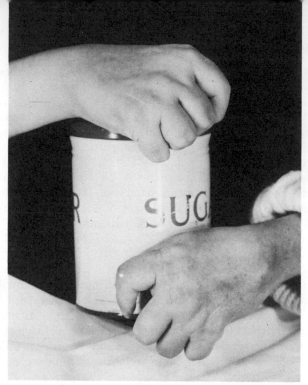

Plate 9/7 Difficulty for deformed fingers is encountered when holding a tin to remove the lid

should familiarise themselves with the general range. They will then be better able to spot the patient who can be helped and if there is no occupational therapist in their hospital they can then contact a therapist attached to the local authority.

Alterations in the Home

Unless the furniture is required for support, it should be moved to provide a clear floor area for walking. The use of crutches and other aids in confined spaces is difficult. Easily held, strong rails should be placed beside all stairs and steps, and banisters should be fitted to both sides of the main house stairs. Rails may also be required outside the house to provide extra support during wet or snowy weather, and this is particularly important if the patient needs to use an outside toilet. For the severely disabled the ideal answer inside the home is to provide a ground-floor bedroom and bathroom, and outside to replace all steps by suitably inclined ramps. For flat dwellers a change of accommodation may be necessary.

Patients with knee or hip joint involvement have difficulty in sitting down and rising from chairs, beds and toilets of the normal height, and this is particularly so if a supporting knee joint splint is used. Appropriate alterations in height can easily be undertaken, but many patients prefer a special chair which is not only of the correct height but which has firm arms, a high moulded back and a seat of reduced depth.

Alterations to a patient's home and the selection of furniture is clearly a personal matter and for the patient to gain the greatest benefit from such changes there must be a close collaboration between the hospital and local authority. Much of the assessment for the detailed work must necessarily be done in a patient's own home, with the combined advice of staff based in the hospital and of domiciliary workers based on the local authority.

Transport and travel may become an increasing problem for the arthritic, and those with a very limited walking ability may be eligible for a mobility allowance. The lists of those eligible for such assistance with outdoor transport is under continuing review and thus if an arthritic patient appears to be eligible for assistance he should be referred to the nearest Department of Health and Social Security appliance centre.

Many patients will require advice in planning a pattern of daily living which is more economical of work output, so that heavier and more difficult tasks are spread over the week. Patients are reluctant to accept that routine tasks such as washing need not be done on fixed days, and that there are different ways of ironing, cooking, etc. They must learn to constantly adjust to their disease, increasing activity slowly, resting as required and enrolling help from the family without feeling that their independence is endangered. The physiotherapist and occupational therapist will find it useful to work together with more disabled patients to practise transfers from bed to chair to toilet, and to plan simple ways of coping with functional problems.

The medical social worker should assess the patient's reaction to the disease, simplify the general explanation, advice and encouragement given by other members of the team, identify any special domestic, social or psychiatric problems, and assist in finding suitable employment. The medical social worker can often discuss, particularly with women, sexual problems created by the disease. However, in many cases this advice is best given by the hospital consultant or the general practitioner. Advice about a change of employment should not be given hurriedly as lighter jobs are usually less well paid. The prognosis in many forms of joint disease is often better than is imagined and the patient should be encouraged to return to his original employment. When the patient is determined on a change of job every help should

be given him. A personal approach to an employer is always worth-
while. Assistance from the Disablement Resettlement Officer may
be required, especially for men, so that arrangements for re-
employment, assessment of employment potential and retraining can
be arranged.

Wheelchairs

At the present time there are more than 100 000 wheelchair users in
the United Kingdom. These chairs are supplied through the Department of Health and Social Security's Artificial Limb and Appliance
Centres (DHSS ALAC), although many patients may be assessed in
hospital clinics with a technical officer from the nearest centre in
attendance. Increasingly, remedial therapists attend such clinics with
their patients, realising that a wheelchair is not a sign of disability but
merely an aid to mobility and that they are often the best people to
advise on the type of chair to be provided.

Clearly an extensive description of wheelchairs is beyond the scope
of this book and those interested should read the Supplement on
wheelchairs in *Equipment for the Disabled*.

In choosing a wheelchair the aims and needs of the patient must be
carefully reviewed and a visit to the patient's home is invaluable. The
chair should increase a patient's mobility and independence, but
unfortunately many chairs are so badly selected that they do neither.
In the same context it is important that a patient should not use all her
energy propelling a chair if an electrically propelled chair would really
allow greater independence. Genuine effort by a patient must be
encouraged but it must not be allowed to become wasteful effort.
(There is a danger that the increased use of the upper limb joints and
the shoulder girdle required to propel a chair leads to an increased rate
of damage in these joints.) The correct assessment of this moment of
transition should dictate the change from walking to using a chair, and
again from using a self-propelled to an electrically propelled chair.

TYPES OF WHEELCHAIRS

Indoor chairs are designed for their ability to be manoeuvred easily in
small spaces, they can be rigid or folding. They are usually self-
propelled by large, 61cm (24in) diameter, front or rear wheels. The
front wheeled type are the more easily handled indoors, especially on
carpets, but the wheels impede side transfers. Rigid outdoor chairs,
designed to be pushed by an attendant, are very comfortable, while
the more commonly used folding chair is ideal for most cars but is
tiring to push for long distances.

Modifications can be made to standard chairs and a range of back-rests, footrests, arms, cushions and brakes is available. Patients should not only be comfortable but able to produce their maximum function.

Electrically powered chairs are available for both indoor and outdoor use and the position and type of control can be modified to suit any patient.

Patients must be instructed in the proper and most efficient manner of using their chair. Too many chairs are unused either due to poor choice on the part of the medical team or due to lack of confidence and ability on the part of the patient.

Technique of making Rest Plasters for the Arm and Leg

LEG

Requirements

A plinth or firm bed with no bottom rail
Two sandbags
Three plastic sheets
4in (10cm), 6in (15cm), 8in (20cm) plaster of Paris slab dispensers
4in (10cm), 6in (15cm) plaster of Paris bandages
A very sharp knife
Plaster scissors
Bottle of oil
Shaving kit for hairy men
Bucket of water (almost cold water in hot weather, warm water in cold weather)
Two small pieces of 2in thick foam (4×6in; 10×15cm)

Method

MEASURE THE PATIENT

Using a tape measure, measure the patient's leg from 1in (2·5cm) below the gluteal fold, down the back of the leg, along the foot extending 2in (5cm) beyond the foot. Add one more inch in ten for shrinkage. Thus if the patient measures 42in (105cm) add 2in to go beyond the foot − 44in + 4½in for shrinkage − 48½in (121·5cm).

Cut the slab to this length. Most patients need 6in (15cm) width slabs. Stout patients need one strip of 8in (20cm) in the middle, with 6in (15cm) width slabs on each side. Three thicknesses of plaster in each layer are required. Roll all the layers.

PREPARE A TROLLEY

For each leg the following is required:

3 rolls of slab
1×6in (15cm) bandage
1×4in (10cm) bandage
1 piece of slab folded for a stirrup for strengthening the heel

PREPARATION OF PATIENT

The patient lies prone with feet beyond the end of the plinth. The foam is placed under each knee lengthways for comfort. A sandbag is placed under each ankle to relax the knees. More sandbags should be used if there is a fixed flexion deformity of the knees, to support the leg at the most straight position that can be obtained without force (Fig. 9/9).

Fig. 9/9 Position of the patient for the making of plaster splints for the leg

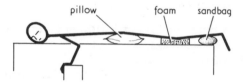

If the knee is very flexed the leg may be gradually straightened as spasm decreases. Wait a little time until this happens. If the knees are very painful it may be necessary for the patient to have a pain relieving injection or tablets a little while beforehand. See that the patient is as comfortable as possible using pillows under the abdomen or head as necessary. The arms may be supported on stools at either side of the plinth.

ORDER OF APPLICATION

a) The first slab goes down the middle of the leg, the second and third to either side
b) The stirrup to reinforce the heel
c) 6in (15cm) bandage crosswise backwards and forwards to reinforce from the top to the back of the knee
d) 4in (10cm) bandage to reinforce the lower leg and cover the stirrup.

Rub each of the layers well in.

FINISHING

Make a mark behind each malleolus; remove the plaster and cut away on the marks.

Trim excess from the leg leaving enough to support the knee laterally; cut excess from the end of the splint.

Put the splint back on to check that it fits properly.

Bind all the edges and cream the inside of the splint to fill small irregularities.

The splints should be dried overnight in a warm place and then bandaged in place for 12 to 24 hours. Check for sore spots and ease plaster if necessary. Then cuff in as follows:

CUFFS FOR LEG PLASTERS

Cuffs are restraining bands of plaster of Paris and should be long enough to go round the leg and the plaster at the appropriate points.

They are 6 layers thick. A piece of Orthoban is placed over the bare skin on the front of the leg in each place, then the slab goes over and around the back of the splint. It should be in good contact but not too tight.

The cuffs are placed:

a) Proximal to the toes
b) Proximal to the ankle joint
c) Distal to the knee joint
d) At the top of the splint covering both top corners.

a), b) and c) are 3in (7·5cm) wide and d) is 4in (10cm) wide. The cuffs take about twenty minutes to dry.

The skin should be cleaned so that little bits of plaster do not fall off and down inside the plaster.

N.B. Plasters are made and cuffed in this way so that all joints may be seen. The joints can then be aspirated, injected or cooled with ice during the time the patient is in the splints, which may be up to three weeks.

ARM

Requirements

Plastic sheet or plinth or table
Bucket of water
Prepared trolley with:

Three rolls of slab – 4in (10cm)

One piece of 4in (10cm) slab folded for a finger cuff (for front of
    fingers)
One rolled bandage
Scissors
Bottle of oil

PREPARATION OF PATIENT

The patient sits sideways at a table with the arm supported. The elbow
is in mid-flexion and the forearm is in pronation with the fingers
resting on a rolled up bandage or small sandbag with the wrist in
mid-position or very slight dorsiflexion. The thumb, which will not
normally be included in the plaster, lies in a position of comfort in
slight flexion.

METHOD

The arm is oiled liberally and the three layers of plaster are then put
on, ending just beyond the fingertips, starting with the middle layer,
and then one each side. Mark round the thumb; take the plaster off
and trim away the excess. Put it back on the patient to check, then
turn the forearm over with the flexor side uppermost and put on the
folded strip, slantwise across the fingers, immediately distal to the
distal interphalangeal joints but not covering the ends of the terminal
phalanges; and around the back of the splint.

   When this has hardened slip the hand out of the splint and bind the
edges and cream the inside.

   When the splints are dry, in about 24 hours, they are bandaged on
to the patient. Next day they can be cuffed into place with bands of
plaster of Paris. These are much more comfortable than bandages.

CUFFS FOR ARM PLASTERS

The finger cuff is already in place. Orthoban is first positioned for
padding and then the other cuffs are placed:

a) Proximal to the wrist joint
b) At the top of the plaster covering both top corners.

BIBLIOGRAPHY

See end of Chapter 12.

Chapter 10

Osteoarthrosis

by C. P. ROBERTS, M.C.S.P. and A. G. MOWAT, M.B., F.R.C.P. (Ed.)

Osteoarthrosis is a disease of synovial joints. In this chapter the involvement of peripheral joints will be considered while the disease as it affects the spine is discussed in Chapter 11. Problems arise over terminology. Although descriptions of the lesions were written as early as 1743, the term osteoarthritis was not used until 1907, after a century during which many researchers had made obvious the differences between it and the other types of arthritis. The absence of obvious inflammation made the purists wish to change the name to osteoarthrosis, although, as we shall see, this is not necessarily correct, while the apparent association of the lesions with ageing has led North American writers in particular to use the term degenerative joint disease. This also may prove to be an incorrect interpretation of the pathology. In this chapter we shall use the term osteoarthrosis. It is characterised by deterioration and disintegration of the articular cartilage and also by the formation of new bone at the articular surfaces. Patients will complain of pain, stiffness and restricted joint movement and will often have bony swelling and joint deformity.

EPIDEMIOLOGY

Osteoarthrosis is a common condition which has affected Man for millions of years. Archaeologists have found evidence of the disease in dinosaurs and in the early remains of human skeletons. Population surveys show the apparent association of the disease with age. Some 10 per cent of patients in their late teens and early 20s have radiographic evidence of the disease and this rises to 70 per cent in patients over the age of 60. However, the incidence of symptoms attributable to these radiographic lesions is much lower, being perhaps 25 per cent in those over the age of 60.

It is commonly supposed that the disease chiefly affects the major weight-bearing joints and is, perhaps, a consequence of man having developed an upright posture. Although such a theory can be supported by the relative increase in symptoms and clinical problems in the hip and knee joints this is only part of the story, since radiographic features are widely spread through most peripheral joints while there is almost complete sparing of the ankle joint from both radiographic and clinical features. Race and geographical location has little effect upon the incidence of the disease although there are local differences which reflect different usage. Thus hip disease is uncommon in the Chinese and Arabs; excessive use of the hands is associated with increased disease, and load carrying on the head, usually by women, is accompanied by increased damage in the cervical spine. Symptoms tend to be less severe in a warm dry climate.

The disease tends to affect joints bilaterally. The incidence is similar in both sexes, although the pattern of damage tends to be different. The age structure of the population in the United Kingdom and the Western World means that there are more female patients than male.

Osteoarthrosis, because it tends to affect older patients than those with rheumatoid arthritis, causes less loss of time from work. However, it imposes a very considerable burden upon a wide range of medical and supportive services and its economical consequences are therefore important.

AETIOLOGY

It has been convenient to classify osteoarthrosis into two main types, primary and secondary. This is an over simplification since there are probably important causative factors in the primary type while the predisposing factors in the secondary type may, in fact, be unimportant. Certainly there are large numbers of patients in whom the cause is obscure. Some of the factors associated with the development of 'secondary' osteoarthrosis are listed in Table I.

Primary

Primary or generalised osteoarthrosis, as its name implies, affects several joints and is typified by the involvement of the distal interphalangeal joints of the fingers with the development of Heberden nodes. Genetic factors are important, a familial incidence being noted particularly in post-menopausal women.

TABLE I CONDITIONS ASSOCIATED WITH OSTEOARTHROSIS

1. Growth Disturbances	Congenital dysplasia of the hip
	Metaphyseal and epiphyseal dysplasia
	Inequality of leg length
	Slipped upper femoral epiphysis
	Chondromalacia patellae
	Osteochondritis dissecans
2. Traumatic	Intra-articular fracture
	Occupational, e.g. miners, footballers
	Joint laxity, e.g. Ehlers-Danlos, Marfan's syndrome
	Amputation
	Poliomyelitis and paraplegia
3. Metabolic	Haemochromatosis
	Ochronosis
	Chondrocalcinosis
	Acromegaly
4. Post-inflammatory	Chronic polyarthritis, e.g. rheumatoid arthritis
	Gout, pseudo-gout
	Septic arthritis
	Haemophilia
5. Avascular disease of bone	Osteochondritis, e.g. Perthe's disease
	Connective tissue diseases, e.g. S.L.E.
	Corticosteroid therapy
	Alcoholism
	Caisson disease
	Haemoglobinopathies, e.g. sickle cell disease
6. Others	Paget's disease
	Neuropathic arthropathy

GROWTH DISTURBANCES

A variety of congenital abnormalities can lead to the mal-development of a joint and the resultant abnormal load bearing appears to lead to the early appearances of osteoarthrosis. The hip joint is most frequently affected but similar problems can occur at other joints e.g. knock knees (genu valgum). The cause of chondromalacia patellae, so common in teenage girls, and osteochondritis dissecans which occurs in both sexes, usually in teenagers, is unknown, but both can predispose to osteoarthrosis. Inequality in leg length, whether 'true' in relation to a growth disturbance in one of several lower limb epiphyses or 'apparent' due to a flexion deformity at the knee or severe scoliosis, may lead to abnormal loading upon the opposite hip and knee and the development of osteoarthrosis usually in the hip.

TRAUMATIC

Fractures and dislocations involving the joint surface may accelerate the development of osteoarthrosis. However, the role of repeated minor trauma has been over-emphasised. Certainly unusual activity, particularly if it subjects the joint to load in an unusual position or produces micro-fractures in the underlying subchondral bone, may pre-dispose to osteoarthrosis. Examples are found in the knees of coal-miners and the elbows and shoulders of pneumatic drillers. In general, extensive use of a joint in a normal fashion does not cause the lesion and thus sportsmen, such as distance runners who may cover 200 or more miles per week, incur no risk of joint damage although they may suffer a number of other problems, particularly muscle and tendon injuries, due to over-use. The well-known problems in footballers reflect the abnormal loading at the knee following meniscectomy or ligamentous damage and the high incidence of ankle fractures.

Extreme joint laxity is associated with rare conditions such as Ehlers-Danlos and Marfan's syndromes and reflects abnormalities in the collagen and elastic tissue of joint capsules and ligaments. Lesser degrees of joint laxity, common in the general population, express themselves as hyper-extensibility at the knee, elbow, thumb and finger joints. (This is often referred to by lay people as being 'double-jointed' although, of course, the joint is normal, just relatively unre-strained.) The joint tends to move through part of its range under poor muscle control and this can lead in later life to the early development of osteoarthrosis. In younger people it may lead to the development of joint effusions e.g. at the knee after extensive use of a trampoline. Properly controlled hypermobility can be an advantage, e.g. in gym-nasts and ballet dancers, while those, particularly women, with Ehlers-Danlos syndrome often use their disease to advantage as acrobatic dancers in night-clubs or as 'elastic ladies' at the fair before premature osteoarthrosis curtails their activities.

Amputation of part or the whole of one leg, perhaps surprisingly, causes little increase in osteoarthrosis in the opposite hip and knee. However, if the upper limbs are used for weight-bearing via crutches following amputation, poliomyelitis or paraplegia, then the consider-able increase in loading across these joints accelerates the develop-ment of osteoarthrotic lesions. Disuse following poliomyelitis, paraplegia and stroke protects a joint from osteoarthrosis.

METABOLIC

Ochronosis is a rare, inherited disease in which an enzyme deficiency leads to the deposition in cartilage of homogentisic acid, a metabolite which causes its degeneration. Cartilage degeneration and early osteoarthrosis also occurs in the iron overload disease, haemochromatosis and is associated with the deposition of calcium and cartilage. There are several recognised causes of chondrocalcinosis, the most common being pyrophosphate arthropathy (see p. 98), and these are related to enzyme inhibition. However it is a frequent and unexplained radiographic finding in the knee, pubic symphysis, shoulders and wrists of elderly patients.

It is fascinating to speculate that there may be many other similar metabolic abnormalities pre-disposing to osteoarthrosis which await discovery by the research biochemist.

A variety of hormonal deficiencies can be associated with musculo-skeletal symptoms but it is not certain that, for instance, diabetes and hypothyroidism precipitate osteoarthrosis. However, excess of growth hormone producing acromegaly is associated with abnormal joint development and growth and an increased incidence of osteoarthrosis.

POST-INFLAMMATORY

Any form of chronic inflammation in a joint will lead to osteoarthrosis and hence many older patients with rheumatoid arthritis present with clinical and radiographic features of two diseases. The association of pyrophosphate crystals in the joint fluid and synovium and early osteoarthrosis is currently under investigation and it may well turn out that this low grade inflammatory lesion is an important cause. Inadequately treated septic arthritis and repeated haemarthrosis in haemophiliacs cause osteoarthrosis.

AVASCULAR DISEASE OF BONE

A number of unrelated diseases can lead to the obliteration of small bone nutrient blood vessels. The circulation to several bony parts seems particularly precarious and the pattern of damage is similar in most of the listed conditions. The femoral head is the usual affected site and the only site in the juvenile condition of Perthe's disease. Other common sites are the medial femoral condyle of the knee, the humeral head and the lunate bone of the wrist. The exact cause of the vessel obstruction is in most cases unknown. In the connective tissue diseases it may well be vasculitis; in those treated with high doses of corticosteroids and in alcoholics, fat emboli; in Caisson disease, which occurs in those working under increased atmospheric pressure in construction projects, and particularly in divers working on North Sea oil installations, gas bubbles; and in the haemoglobinopathies, plugs of haemolysed red cells.

DIETARY FACTORS

The only known dietary factor causing osteoarthrosis is the eating of fungus-contaminated grain which causes Kashin-Beck disease in young children in Eastern Siberia and Northern China.

Obesity has not been clearly indicated in the causation of osteo-arthrosis. Although overweight patients with osteoarthrosis are urged to diet, this is not always followed by improvement in their symptoms although such weight reduction would be associated with other benefits, not least the ability to co-operate better with the physiotherap-ist and the greater ease and safety of any planned operative treatment.

PATHOLOGY

Osteoarthrosis is primarily a disease of joint cartilage, but as the disease progresses, the capsule, synovial membrane and bone become involved. It is not a systemic disease as is rheumatoid arthritis, in that only the joints are affected, but by virtue of the symptoms caused, the patient may well feel depressed and lethargic. All the listed causes lead to the same pathological features since the end result of abnormal loading, inflammation and metabolic factors is impaired nutrition and repair of cartilage.

The earliest pathological change occurs in the articular cartilage which loses its normal, smooth, glistening appearance, becoming velvety in texture with yellow-brown areas over the surface. It also becomes softened, therefore losing its normal resilience. Flaking and fibrillation of the cartilage occurs and with the appearance of fissures of varying depth, the surface becomes very irregular. The subchon-dral blood vessels hypertrophy, proliferate and invade the cartilage, leading to calcification and eventual ossification. With continued softening, erosion and ulceration, the bone ends become denuded of cartilage and exposed. Continual friction between the opposing joint surfaces produces hardening of the bone which becomes polished, or eburnated. Subchondral cyst formation may be caused by micro-fractures of the trabeculae, resulting from re-alignment of the joint with changed lines of stress, or by the synovial fluid being forced, under pressure, through minute defects in the diseased cartilage.

At any point in the disease process, though usually at a later stage, there may be new bone formation. This can either be minor lipping at joint margins or the development of large osteophytes, which can also be seen at the point of the capsule or ligamentous attachments. Osteophytes are abnormal outgrowths of cancellous bone, often covered by hyaline cartilage. Loose bodies, in the form of flakes of cartilage, are also found and these may sometimes be ossified. Collapse of the articular cartilage and bony surfaces may occur and can progress very rapidly, leading to the eventual disintegration of the whole joint. Fibrosis of the joint capsule and synovial membrane proliferation will produce a thickened joint with a consequent decrease in range of motion. Bony ankylosis occasionally occurs.

Throughout the course of the disease, bone remodelling will take place, minor in the early stages, but often considerable later on. This remodelling alters the normal lines of force through the joint, thus adding to the ever increasing deformity.

Radiographic Changes

Radiographic evidence of degenerative changes can be misleading as they do not always correlate with the patient's symptoms. A patient with severe symptoms may only have minor radiographic changes, while sometimes quite marked changes give rise to no complaints at all. The radiographic features that may be seen are:

1. Diminished joint space due to cartilage loss (more noticeable in weight-bearing pictures)
2. Sclerosis of subchondral bone
3. Subchondral bone cysts
4. Osteophyte formation at joint margins
5. Irregularities of joint surfaces
6. Loose bodies
7. Collapse of subchondral bone
8. Subluxation with resulting mal-alignment of joint
9. Bony ankylosis.

Laboratory Findings

There are really no laboratory tests of value in the diagnosis of osteoarthrosis. A variety of tests may support one or other of the possible 'secondary' causes and suggest a possible line of treatment for the underlying disease. Although inflammatory mechanisms may be important this is rarely reflected in routine tests. Thus the ESR is normal or minimally elevated and the rheumatoid factor tests show only the expected low incidence of positivity found in a normal population. The synovial fluid is clear and yellow, has normal viscosity and a low cell count.

SIGNS AND SYMPTOMS

The symptoms which a patient describes often reflect the stage to which the disease has progressed, but occasionally it is not possible to correlate a patient's story of severe pain and disability with the examination and radiographic findings.

The disease course tends to be progressive and chronic with exacerbations, sometimes related to trauma, although it can be rapidly downward.

Pain

Pain is the principal feature of osteoarthrosis although a few patients will mention only stiffness. Complaints reflecting limited movement are common although these often have to be established by direct questioning and examination. Pain is of several different types:

a) *Immobility pain*. Pain and stiffness after periods of inactivity and on rising in the morning is due to thickening of capsular structures. The duration and severity is much less than that which accompanies inflammatory joint disease and rarely persists for more than 10 to 15 minutes.

b) *Pain on weight bearing*. This is due to abnormal joint loading and the roughened surfaces, and is exaggerated by deformity.

c) *Pain on movement*. This is due to movement across a roughened surface but is also caused by capsular tightness and disuse of the full range of movement.

d) *Night pain*. Night pain sufficient to waken the patient is a characteristic feature of osteoarthrosis and is often an indication of the severity of the damage. It is probably due to abnormal venous congestion in the subchondral bone and the success of some surgical procedures, particularly osteotomy, is partly due to the correction of this congestion. Simple vascular decompression by the insertion of valved drains has recently been shown to be effective in the relief of night pain.

e) *Pain of inflammation*. Possible inflammatory mechanisms have been discussed under causation.

f) *Pain of trauma*. Continuation of the initiating traumatic process or any sudden increase in joint loading will cause pain. This type of pain is probably the only one that can be modified by a change in the patient's pattern of activity.

g) *Psychological pain*. Pain from an osteoarthrotic joint can be aggravated or largely caused by psychological factors. Reduced activity which most patients find difficult to accept undoubtedly causes stress and this in turn can exacerbate the symptoms and disability. Patients undoubtedly have very variable pain thresholds and this partly explains the discrepancy between clinical and radiographic features.

h) *Referred pain.* Pain from joint structures, particularly capsules and ligaments which are richly supplied with nerve endings, may be referred to any point in the same dermatome. Referred pain of sufficient severity and duration may lead to the development of a clinically misleading referred tender spot. A full clinical examination, a consideration of the innervation of joint structures in relation to the diagrams of skin dermatomes on p. 154 and an appreciation that the pain could not be arising from any structure at the point of tenderness will lead to the correct diagnosis. The most typical example of referred pain is that between the hip and knee joints. The patients may feel all their pain in the wrong joint and be surprised at and reluctant to accept the correct interpretation.

As the range of joint motion lessens, muscles acting on the joint will not work to their full capacity and will therefore weaken and atrophy. General muscle weakness of a limb with associated loss of function will often follow, as the joints are interdependent on one another for full function to be achieved. Thus limited movement in the knee and ankle may result from hip disease.

Protective muscle spasm is the body's attempt to limit joint movement and so reduce pain to a minimum.

Joint Deformity

The deformities are the result of the pathological changes previously described. Alteration in articular surface alignment, as in valgus or varus deformities of the knee, will give one type of appearance, while muscle imbalance between for example, the hamstrings and weak quadriceps muscles will give a fixed flexion deformity. Heberden's nodes are a characteristic deforming influence on the distal interphalangeal joints of the fingers (Plate 10/1).

Joint Appearance

Osteoarthrotic joints are often enlarged due to new bone and osteophyte formation, or synovial and capsular thickening. Moderate effusions may be seen, usually associated with an acute episode.

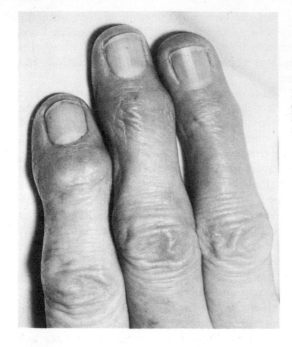

Plate 10/1 Generalised
osteoarthrosis of the
hand showing Heberden
node formation

Crepitus

This is an easily felt fine or coarse grating of opposing irregular joint
surfaces. In the later stages, when bone ends are in direct contact,
joint movement may become jerky with a loud 'clunking', easily heard
a few yards away.

Loss of Function

This is the most important sign, as it is the accumulative result of the
disease process leading, if left untreated, to eventual loss of independence and often loss of self-respect. Patients will often volunteer some
aspects such as a decreased walking distance, difficulty in climbing
stairs or standing for long periods. However, many will need to be
taken through, verbally, a typical day's activities to determine the
extent of their disability. Shame and loss of self-respect may still mean
they fail to describe the full extent of their disability, particularly in
relation to aspects of personal hygiene. Thus direct examination of a
wide range of activities, which can often be usefully done with the
occupational therapist is important. Further, questioning of a spouse
or relative, particularly about activities it is difficult to test, such as

transport difficulties, reluctance to go shopping or visit friends is also important. The examination with the occupational therapist can lead to a sensible, combined therapeutic approach.

CLINICAL FEATURES

Patients will complain of pain, loss of function, stiffness and sometimes of instability, the latter particularly if the knee is involved. Changes in the weather appear to influence symptoms, being more severe when it is cold and damp. Initially, loss of function is related to pain and resultant muscle spasm, but at a later stage this is superseded by joint deformity and muscle weakness.

Hip

Pain is felt in the groin, over the greater trochanter, over the anterior aspect of the thigh and in the knee, the latter occasionally being the only painful area. Both hips are usually affected, although one may be in advance of the other (Plate 10/2). A reduction in active and passive movements occurs gradually with the joint taking up the typical deformity of flexion, adduction and lateral rotation. This tendency is often accelerated by spasm of the muscles producing those movements. Inequality of leg length is a frequent finding, 'apparent' shortening being due to the pelvis being raised on the affected side, in an attempt to keep the leg vertical, and 'true' shortening the result of femoral head or neck collapse and deformity or protrusio acetabuli. A compensatory lumbar lordosis may cause low back pain and the lateral tilt of the pelvis may produce a scoliosis. Trendelenburg's sign is often

Plate 10/2 Radiograph of bilateral osteoarthrosis of the hips, showing the diminished joint space, cystic changes, sclerosis and osteophyte formation

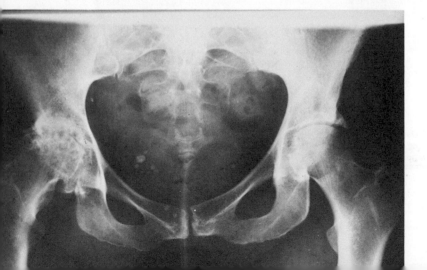

positive, being due to gluteus medius weakness (Plates 10/3 and 10/4). This, together with a fixed deformity and pain, will produce a limp, which can be made less obvious if a stick is used in the opposite hand.

Disability mainly results from loss of flexion and difficulties will include:

    i)   Putting on socks and shoes
    ii) Cutting toe-nails
    iii) Sitting or rising from bed, chair and toilet

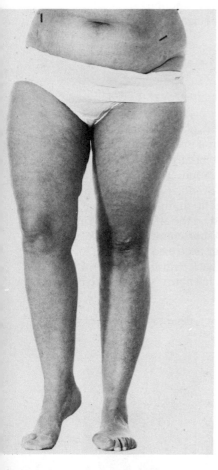 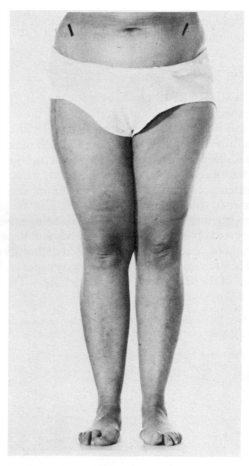

Plate 10/3 Osteoarthrosis of the right hip showing how the pelvis is tilted on the right to compensate for the adduction deformity

Plate 10/4 Following arthroplasty, the same patient as Plate 10/3 is shown with the adduction deformity corrected

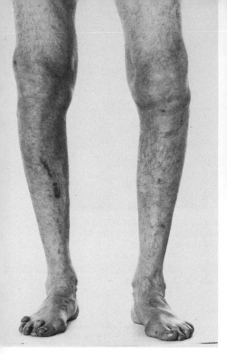

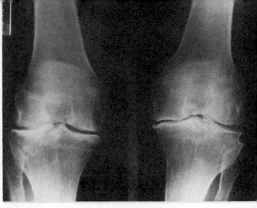

Plate 10/5 (*left*) Bilateral osteoarthrosis of the knees showing varus deformity

Plate 10/6 (*above*) Radiographs of the knee joints of the patient in Plate 10/5

iv) Sitting up in bed
v) Climbing stairs
vi) Getting into and out of a bath

Walking distance will be reduced. Patients can rarely give distances and need familiar landmarks to measure distances such as to the local shop, to the Post Office for pensions, the pub, bus stop, etc. Precise distances are less important than an interpretation of the meaning of the disability upon independence and an assessment of what form of treatment might again bring these places to within the patient's range.

Knee

Pain is around the joint, often over one compartment more than the other; stiffness after rest and instability, especially when negotiating stairs or rough ground, are the common complaints. There may be a moderate effusion and some tenderness around the joint margins can often be elicited. The joint may be enlarged, often with a varus, valgus or flexion deformity, accentuated by weight-bearing (Plates 10/5, 10/6, 10/7, 10/8). Full range of movement is lost and crepitus in both joint compartments and between patella and femur is a common finding. In young people pain and patello-femoral crepitus with a full range of movement, is often chondromalacia patellae and not true osteoarthritis. The patient may walk with a limp and have apparent

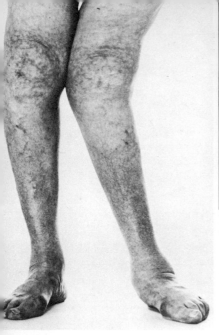

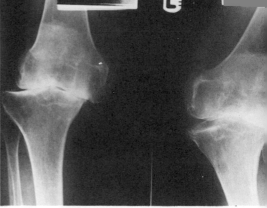

Plate 10/7 (*left*) Bilateral osteoarthrosis of the knees showing gross valgus deformity of the left knee and subluxation of the right

Plate 10/8 (*above*) Radiographs of the knee joints of the patient in Plate 10/7

shortening of the leg, but this will be due to a varus, valgus or flexion deformity. The knee will flex during the swing through phase of walking as compared to a rheumatoid patient who will hold the knee still so as to avoid the pain caused by stretching the inflamed periarticular structures.

Locking of the joint due to severe joint surface damage, the presence of a loose body or a damaged meniscus is a very common feature in the knee joint. The knee, more than most joints, is dependent upon good muscle control and ligamentous integrity for stability, as the joint surfaces convey little natural stability. Thus muscle weakness and ligamentous damage may cause distressing instability with a feeling of unreliability and a tendency for the joint to 'give way' in the presence of only moderate joint changes. However, if untreated, these factors will lead rapidly to osteoarthrotic changes.

Foot

The first metatarsophalangeal (MTP) joint of the foot is the most commonly affected joint, occurring in young adults and in men more than women. Disease at this joint is called hallux rigidus. The patient will complain of pain, often severe, increased by walking. The symptoms are reduced by wearing thick-soled shoes/boots, so limiting joint movement. Hyperextension of the interphalangeal joint develops to compensate for the loss of MTP joint extension. Osteoarthrosis in the ankle and other foot joints is rare and is usually secondary to trauma and inflammatory disease.

Hand

A variety of patterns of disease may be present, but the most characteristic is that associated with primary osteoarthrosis. The most obvious features are Heberden nodes which may affect any or all of the distal interphalangeal joints of the fingers and the interphalangeal

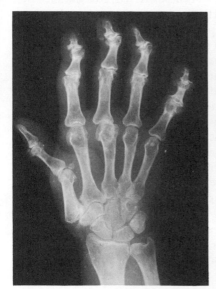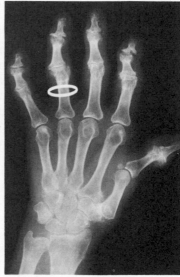

Plate 10/9 Radiograph of generalised osteoarthrosis of the hands showing Heberden nodes on the distal interphalangeal joints, Bouchard's nodes on the proximal interphalangeal joints and the adducted thumbs due to arthritis in the first carpo-metacarpal joints

joint of the thumb, usually symmetrically (Plate 10/9). These nodes are essentially a product of the exuberant osteophytes from both sides of the joint margin. They are usually painless but acute, exacerbations of the osteoarthrotic process may produce severe pain and a red, hot, swollen and tender cystic enlargement of the node which settles over one to two weeks. Disease of the proximal interphalangeal joints, although less common, follows a similar pattern, the deformities being called Bouchard's nodes. The lesions are cosmetically unattractive and often the fairly rapid change in a middle-aged woman's hand appearance over perhaps three to five years can be very distressing. In

addition, flexion and lateral deformity, particularly at the distal interphalangeal joints, tends to make the fingers rather clumsy.

The clinical features and symptoms are clearly related to trauma
even if genetic factors are important. The dominant hand is worst
affected and signs often appear first and are exaggerated in a joint that
has been the site of previous trauma. The involvement of one or two
joints in men can usually be clearly related to trauma. Many female
patients tend to be vigorous hand users, being keen sewers, gardeners,
etc.

Symptomatic treatment is all that can be offered. Reassurance that
they do not have rheumatoid arthritis is important, together with
advice about hand usage. Heat, particularly wax treatment, may be
helpful. Surgical treatment, with fusion of the distal interphalangeal
joint in 10° of flexion and the proximal interphalangeal joint in 45° of
flexion is occasionally carried out.

Metacarpophalangeal joint disease is uncommon, usually affecting
the index and middle fingers in men. Inflammatory episodes in these
joints frequently suggest a diagnosis of rheumatoid arthritis.

Involvement of the carpo-metacarpal joint of the thumb is common
in both sexes, being part of the pattern of primary generalised osteoarthrosis in women. The pain, crepitus and adduction deformity is
associated with decreased opposition of the thumb to the fingers and
secondary wasting of the muscles of the thenar eminence. The overall
appearance is of a 'square hand'.

Osteoarthrosis is uncommon at the *wrist*, except as a result of
trauma of a Colles fracture. However, often very minor changes may
produce median nerve compression symptoms without pain or any
limitation in joint movement.

In the other peripheral joints, osteoarthrosis usually occurs as a
result of previous trauma. Pain is felt around the joint with limitation
of movement. In the shoulder, reduced rotation is the most debilitating sign and an occasional complication at the elbow is entrapment of
the ulnar nerve.

Acromioclavicular, sternoclavicular and costovertebral joints are
commonly involved, pain being felt over the joint.

Osteoarthrosis in the synovial joints of the *spine* is discussed in
Chapter 11.

PHYSIOTHERAPY

Patients with varying degrees of osteoarthrotic change are referred to
physiotherapy departments for treatment. However severe the signs

and symptoms are, a careful examination is essential to aid the choice of treatment prior to its initiation.

Examination

The patient's notes should be read and any relevant information recorded. Occupation, likely exacerbating activities, social background and radiographic findings are important points to note.

By questioning the patient, the severity, position and nature of the pain as described earlier can be elicited and the degree of stiffness judged. More importantly, the amount of functional disability involved can be discovered. An assessment of the patient's likely co-operation in any planned treatment programme must be made, while the therapist must set realistic goals for herself and the patient. All too often the patient will have unrealistic expectations and hence be disappointed. Indeed, in some patients the expectations and wishes may be so unrealistic that no treatment should be given. Thus a desire to be able to climb the stairs again may be beyond the ability of any treatment to satisfy and the therapist's energies are better channelled into persuading the patient of the wisdom and advantages of living downstairs or considering alternative accommodation. It cannot be emphasised too strongly that a detailed functional assessment must be undertaken before starting treatment. Difficulties relating to work or hobbies should be noted as these are usually of great concern to the patient. An ability to perform normal activities is a good guide to the efficacy of treatment.

Lastly, with out-patients the details of how they propose to reach the department must be determined. All are aware that lengthy ambulance journeys for short periods of largely passive therapy are worthless unless it is accepted that social contact is the only point of the exercise.

Unobtrusive observation of the patient, noting gait, ease or otherwise of dressing and the use of trick movements and aids is important, as there is sometimes a discrepancy between the patient's stated functional problems and those actually observed. The size and shape of the joint, the presence of deformity, muscle wasting and the position in which the limb is held, are noted and a comparison made with the other limb.

Palpation for temperature, bony enlargement, tenderness, effusion, soft tissue thickening, and, on passive movement, crepitus, should be carried out where possible.

Movements, both active and passive, should be tested, measured accurately and recorded, with any discrepancy between the two limbs noted. Care must be taken when testing passive range to ensure that only movement at one joint is performed. If range of movement is limited, a reason should be sought. Is it pain, muscle weakness, muscle spasm, joint stiffness, bony block or some other reason?

Instability due to ligamentous laxity should be tested for.

Muscle power needs to be checked and graded and compared with the other limb.

Leg length should be measured for 'true' and 'apparent' shortening. 'True' shortening is measured from the anterior superior iliac spine to the medial malleolus, and 'apparent' shortening from the umbilicus or xiphisternum to the medial malleolus. This is important as a patient's mobility can be greatly improved by the provision of a shoe raise if this should be found necessary.

A brief examination of the joints above and below the one of particular interest is important, as full function is dependent on all the joints in a limb working effectively.

Treatment

The principal aim for the physiotherapist is to give the patient maximum independence. This may be achieved by:

a) reducing pain, often of primary importance to the patient
b) improving joint movement

PAIN RELIEF

Ice packs or towels will ease pain and reduce effusions when placed over the joint for up to 30 minutes. The skin condition should be noted, as it is just as possible to get a burn from ice as it is from heat; a patient with sensitive skin should not have ice applied for very long periods. Hands and feet are more easily treated in an ice bath. Exercise during ice treatment should be encouraged and it is often found to be easier (see p. 106).

Heat in any of its forms can be given to reduce pain and muscle spasm, but it is purely symptomatic and rarely gives any lasting benefit if given by itself. Its primary function is to improve the patient's ability to perform her exercises.

Ultrasound can be used to reduce pain over localised tender areas, around the joints.

Hydrotherapy is useful where there is more than one joint needing treatment, as with lumbar spine involvement, or where an attempt at ambulation is to be made with a previously chairbound patient. It can also be useful when a particularly nervous individual is to be treated (see p. 107).

Drug treatment is described in Chapter 15.

INCREASED RANGE OF MOTION

Any increase in range of motion must be accompanied by an increase in muscle power, so that control over the joint throughout the range is achieved.

Muscle spasm must be reduced as quickly as possible before it becomes established and fixed deformities develop. Hydrotherapy, sling suspension and ice towels placed along the length of the muscle, combined with exercise can be used to this end. Muscle relaxation using such techniques as 'hold relax' and 'slow reversal relax' can be used. Prolonged stretching of the muscle group in spasm can aid that muscle's relaxation.

Tight structures around the joint, such as the capsule and ligaments, must be eased for any increase in movement to be achieved. Passive mobilisation as described by Maitland (1977) is extremely valuable but must be carefully graded. Sling suspension and slippery board exercises will increase range by the use of repetitive movements to the limit of the available range. Hydrotherapy and traction, either manual or mechanical, will also increase movement, especially in the hip and spine.

Muscle strength must be increased to enable the patient to take full advantage of any lessening of symptoms. A full passive range of motion with no pain is of no functional value if the patient cannot control the joint. Appropriate exercises are therefore essential to build up muscle power at the same rate as any increased range of movement is achieved.

Simple exercises, gravity, spring, weight or manually resisted, must not be overlooked, as excellent results are obtained. Straight-forward straight leg raising exercises are effective for the knee and are relatively easy for the patient to perform at home. Slings and pulleys are useful when muscles are very weak and the principle of inclined planes can be utilised with the slippery board. Hydrotherapy can be used, water providing the resistance, which can be increased by using floats and flippers. Proprioceptive neuromuscular facilitation techniques can be used to increase both muscle power and range of movement. These are sometimes preferred as they are functional and have a rotary component, but they are time-consuming to perform, which is often a critical factor governing the choice of exercises in a busy department.

Functional Re-education

With decreasing pain and increasing joint mobility and control, emphasis in treatment must be placed more and more on functional activities, although some re-training in daily living activities must be incorporated at all stages of the treatment programme. Patients with lower limb osteoarthrosis may require training in sitting from lying or standing, turning and getting out of bed, standing from sitting, climbing stairs and getting in or out of a car or bus.

Gait training is important and use can be made initially of the pool and/or parallel bars. A mirror at the end of the bars enables the physiotherapist to point out faults and encourages the patient not to look at his feet, with consequent improvement in his posture. Sticks and elbow crutches and, in the face of severe disease, gutter crutches or walking frames, are used to preserve the joints and alleviate symptoms as far as possible. If the shoulders are involved, the minimum of walking aids should be used. A shoe raise is beneficial if there is shortening of one leg. Patients usually find climbing stairs easier if the non-affected leg goes up first and down last.

Continued exercises at home are vitally important if any improvement gained by treatment is to be lasting. A simple exercise regime should be taught when the patient is first seen, to be carried out between supervised sessions, and perhaps more importantly, after treatment has ended, so that ground gained can be maintained. To exercise through pain is not a good thing, especially during an acute attack, and this should be emphasised to the patient. Those with osteoarthrosis of the hip should be told to spend at least one hour a day lying prone with the legs as far apart as possible, as this will help in preventing deformities by stretching the flexors and adductors.

Advice on the amount of activity that should be undertaken and on simple changes of life style that may be helpful should be given at an early stage. For example, a high stool can be used to rest the legs when washing-up or ironing. If full independence is not achieved, a whole range of aids and house adaptions can be used to ease the problems. Advice from an occupational therapist at this point is very valuable and a visit to the patient's own home is occasionally indicated as a better assessment of the problems can be made in the patient's own environment.

Dietary Advice

Although many osteoarthrotic patients are overweight the contribution of this in the causation of the disease is disputed, while there is little evidence that weight reduction in itself leads to a decrease in symptoms. Nevertheless, patients are often told to lose one or two stone in weight before the surgeon will consider operating and in the meantime they should attend the physiotherapy department. Although such an approach is to be deplored, altering the practice is often difficult! Certainly the overweight patient is less able to co-operate with the therapist. If weight reduction is considered important either for operative safety reasons or to facilitate pre- and postoperative physiotherapy then proper dietary advice and support must be sought. Although the personal contact between the therapist and patient can be used to encourage weight reduction, without adequate help from a dietician it is an abuse of the therapist's time and skills.

Treatment must be tailored to the individual patient and will depend on the stage of the disease, age, and her ability to understand and follow instructions. Of primary importance is a desire on the part of the patient to get better, as if this is lacking, little or no progress will be possible.

A stage will be reached when, in the opinion of the physician and therapist, the benefits of further treatment will be minimal, and it is at this point that surgical intervention will be considered.

REFERENCE

Maitland, G. D., (1977). *Peripheral Manipulation*, 2nd edition. Butterworths.

BIBLIOGRAPHY

See end of Chapter 12.

ACKNOWLEDGEMENT

Plates 10/3, 10/4, 10/5, 10/6, 10/7, 10/8 and 10/9 were previously used in the 5th edition in the chapter written by Miss B. Graveling, M.C.S.P. The authors are grateful to Miss Graveling for kindly agreeing to their use in this new chapter.

Chapter 11

Degenerative Arthritis of the Spine and Intervertebral Disc Disease

by A. G. MOWAT, M.B., F.R.C.P. (Ed.)
and J. M. ABERY, M.C.S.P.

ANATOMY, PATHOLOGY, INCIDENCE AND CAUSE

The Spinal Apophyseal Joints

The spinal apophyseal joints are diarthrodial, synovial joints and are thus susceptible to be involved in the same inflammatory and degenerative processes which affect larger, peripheral joints. The apophyseal joints lie posteriorly on each side of the vertebral pedicles providing articulation with the adjacent vertebrae, and so each vertebra carries four articular surfaces (Plate 11/1). In addition each thoracic vertebra has four small articular surfaces for the articulation of the ribs with the sides of the vertebral body and the transverse processes. The atlas and axis (the first and second cervical vertebrae) carry similar posterior apophyseal joints, but in addition there are synovial joints between the anterior arch of the atlas and the odontoid process of the axis. The third to the seventh cervical vertebral bodies differ from those elsewhere in the spine in having small synovial joints on the posterior edge of the upper and lower surfaces of the bodies – neuro-central joints.

The spinal movements which take place at each vertebra are flexion, extension, lateral flexion and rotation, the latter two being associated movements. The extent of these movements at each part of the spine depends upon the thickness of the intervertebral discs, the tension in the interspinal ligaments and the angle of contact of the intervertebral joints. In consequence, greater movements occur in the cervical and lumbar spine than in the thoracic spine and for practical purposes none occurs in the sacral region. The joints between the atlas and the skull allow flexion, extension and lateral flexion of the skull

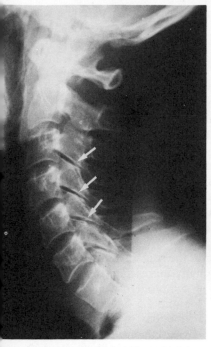

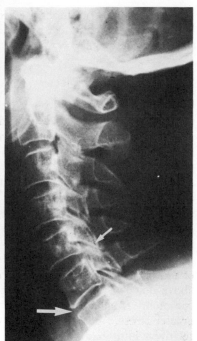

Plate 11/1 A normal lateral radiograph of the cervical spine showing that the intervertebral discs are well-preserved with little evidence of osteophyte formation on the anterior or posterior margins of the vertebral bodies. The apophyseal joints (arrowed) are normal

Plate 11/2 A lateral radiograph of the cervical spine showing narrowing of the C6–7 disc and apophyseal joint arthritis

while rotation of the skull upon the cervical spine is almost entirely carried out by the axis.

Degenerative arthritis in these joints, with loss of cartilage, eburnation of underlying bone and the development of marginal osteophytes, accompanied by a very variable amount of pain and decreased function, is a very common feature of advancing age (Plate 11/2). Surveys based upon radiographic findings show that some 70 per cent of the population has such changes by the age of 60 years and that the incidence steadily increases with age. Occupational factors tend to affect the incidence, since degenerative changes are commoner in men, particularly those engaged in manual work. Further, the incidence especially of cervical spinal lesions, is exaggerated in those patients, mostly women, with primary generalised osteoarthrosis with Heberden nodes around the distal interphalangeal joints of the hands.

However, it must be emphasised that there is no correlation between the radiographic findings and the presence or severity of clinical symptoms and signs.

The Intervertebral Discs

The intervertebral discs, lying between successive vertebral bodies from the second cervical vertebra downwards, are composed of fibro-cartilage, the outer portion of which consists chiefly of concentric rings of fibrous tissue, the annulus fibrosus, while the centre of the disc, the nucleus pulposus, is softer and gelatinous. The normal disc is capable of withstanding heavy loads with relatively little deformation and serves as an efficient 'shock absorber'. It can adapt to spinal movements and should distribute rapidly changing stresses evenly up and down the spine. Recent work suggests that many spines fail to achieve even distribution of stresses.

The discs account for one-quarter of the spinal length, and are not of uniform thickness, being of gradually increasing thickness from above downwards. The frequency of symptoms, which arise most commonly from the C5–6, C6–7, L4–5 and L5–S1 discs, is due to greater stresses being present at the junctions of very mobile and relatively immobile spinal segments. By early adult life the discs are avascular and degenerative changes set in accompanied by a progressive reduction in water content. Such degenerative changes are accompanied by a tendency for the contents of the nucleus pulposus to be extruded through weakened portions of the annulus fibrosus. Such extrusion may occur through the vertebral plate into adjacent vertebrae. These Schmorl's nodes are usually symptomless, but if multiple may be associated with degenerative arthritis and a loss of height.

Extrusion of the disc in other directions is influenced by the attachment of the disc to the vertebral ligaments. The disc is loosely attached to the anterior longitudinal ligament which in turn is firmly attached to the vertebral bodies, but the disc is more firmly attached to the posterior longitudinal ligament which in its turn is only loosely attached to the posterior aspect of the vertebral bodies. Extrusion of the disc anteriorly or laterally causes anterior or lateral osteophyte growth which may be so marked as occasionally to unite and so fuse two vertebrae with consequent loss of movement of the apophyseal joints (Plate 11/3). Extrusion of the disc contents posteriorly causes greater problems. Fixation to the posterior ligament usually means that disc extrusion occurs postero-laterally, at which site symptoms will depend upon whether the extrusion is acute or whether it occurs slowly and is accompanied by osteophyte formation. In either event the disc contents and/or the osteophytes may press upon the spinal cord, the nerve roots either as they travel downwards or through the intervertebral foramina, or upon the vertebral artery in the cervical spine.

The phenomenon of disc degeneration, with or without osteophyte formation and extrusion of disc contents is very common, with 60 per cent of the population having significant radiological changes in all

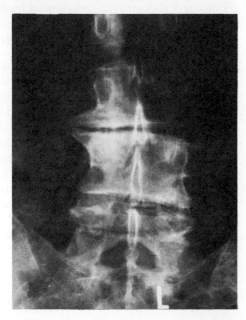

Plate 11/3 Radiograph of lumbar spine showing how antero-lateral osteophytes from adjacent vertebrae have united. Note the associated disc degeneration and narrowing

spinal segments by the age of 60 years. The incidence in all spinal segments is higher in men. Degeneration of discs is often associated with degeneration in the apophyseal joints and once again the radiographic and clinical presentations cannot be correlated (see Plate 11/2).

The incidence of acute disc prolapse, commonest in the lumbar spine and which tends to occur in patients aged between 30 and 50 years, is difficult to determine, since the diagnosis of 'slipped disc' is a fashionable one, particularly by patients. Although acute disc prolapse produces a characteristic clinical picture, the diagnosis is medically proven relatively rarely.

Ligaments and Muscles

As with joint disease elsewhere, there may be related or independent symptoms arising from associated muscles and ligaments. In addition to the anterior and posterior longitudinal ligaments, there are a variety of other spinal ligaments, the most important of which are the ligamentum flava connecting the laminae of adjacent vertebrae, and the interspinous ligaments joining the vertebral spines. A large number of muscles are attached to the spinal column, and these attachments may be the site of chronic inflammation secondary to trauma and abnormal or unbalanced loading.

THE CAUSES OF DEGENERATION IN THE SPINE

The causes of degenerative changes in the spine, sometimes called spondylosis, as with degenerative arthritis in other joints, are not clearly determined. In some patients the association with trauma, either as a single severe episode or related to repeated minor episodes over many years, usually determined by the nature of or the posture adopted at work, will be clear. In others obesity may be a major factor. However, in many patients the cause is unclear although developmental abnormalities and endocrine and metabolic factors may be involved. In the group of patients with widespread generalised osteo-arthrosis genetic factors are dominant, the inheritance among female members of the family often being clearly seen. It is obvious, therefore, that only some of the potential causes can be influenced during management of the patient.

CERVICAL SPINE

Clinical Features

Three main groups of symptoms are produced by degenerative arthritis and intervertebral disc disease in the cervical spine. (a) Symptoms due to pressure of osteophytes or postero-lateral disc protrusion on the spinal nerves. These are by far the commonest symptoms. (b) Symptoms due to pressure of osteophytes or central disc protrusion on the spinal cord. (c) Symptoms due to pressure of osteophytes or lateral disc protrusion on the vertebral artery (Plates 11/4 and 11/5).

Degeneration in the neuro-central joints of the third to seventh vertebrae may contribute to both spinal cord and nerve compression.

Symptoms may be produced by acute or chronic disc changes. Acute disc prolapse usually follows trauma in younger patients and produces sudden severe pain with a further increase in intensity over a few days. Changes associated with chronic disc disease are more gradual and frequently episodic in their production of symptoms.

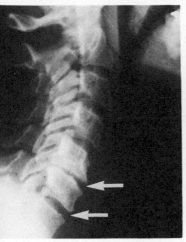

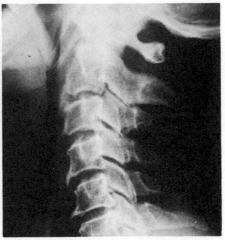

Plate 11/4 A lateral radiograph of the cervical spine showing narrowing of the C5–6 and C6–7 discs with anterior and posterior osteophyte formation (arrowed). The apophyseal joints are well-preserved

Plate 11/5 A lateral radiograph of the cervical spine showing marked osteophyte formation

SPINAL NERVE ROOT COMPRESSION

Spinal nerve root compression produces pain in the distribution area of the root, but it is important to remember that the pain may be wider spread than imagined, with C4 root pain being felt in the scapular region and C7 root pain in the anterior chest. Typically, acute spasms of pain are added to a background of dull aching. The pain may produce muscle spasm with a reduction in spinal movement or a complete loss of movement associated with a torticollis. Involvement of the motor root results in muscle weakness and diminution or absence of arm reflexes. The muscles supplied by the most commonly involved roots are listed below:

Deltoid	C5, (6)
Biceps	C(5), 6
Triceps	C(6), 7, (8)
Wrist and fingers extensors and flexors	C7, 8
Thumb abductors and extensors	C(7), 8
Intrinsic hand muscles	C8, T1

Involvement of the sensory root may produce paraesthesiae and subsequently impairment of all modalities of sensation in the affected dermatome. In the early stages, nerve root irritation may produce increased and unpleasant sensation – hyperaesthesia. Skin dermatomes are shown in Fig. 11/1, but caution must be exercised in attributing symptoms to a specific root on the basis of such diagrams, as there is marked individual variation.

CERVICAL SPINAL CORD COMPRESSION

Cervical spinal cord compression is a very serious condition which occurs most commonly at the C5–6 level. Although there is a variety of presentations, the most usual involves upper motor neurone lesion findings in one or both legs with lower motor neurone lesion findings in the upper limbs. In addition there will be a variety of sensory abnormalities in both arms and legs.

VERTEBRAL ARTERY COMPRESSION

Vertebral artery compression can lead, particularly in the elderly, to brain stem ischaemia and the production of vertigo, tinnitus, visual disturbances, difficulty with speech and swallowing, and ataxia and other signs of cerebellar dysfunction.

Involvement of individual spinal joints or muscle and ligamentous damage in the neck, may produce both local and referred pain often

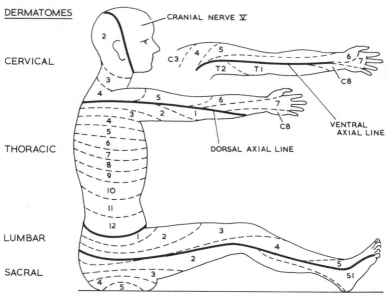

Fig. 11/1 Plan of the dermatomes of the body and the segmental cutaneous distribution of the upper limb

associated with secondary muscle spasm, reduced movement and torticollis. Such symptoms are the usual result of 'whiplash' injuries incurred in road traffic accidents. The particular problems associated with disease of the atlanto-axial joints have been described elsewhere (see Chapter 6).

INVESTIGATION AND TREATMENT OF CERVICAL SPINE LESIONS

The physiotherapist has an important role in the assessment of patients with cervical spinal disease. An accurate history will often pinpoint the lesion and diagnosis, and an assessment of the patient's response to pain and disability will provide useful information in judging the severity of the symptoms and the patient's likely response to treatment. In particular, if a patient's reaction is not to be misjudged, it must be remembered that symptoms bear little or no relationship to radiographic features.

It is vital that the physiotherapist undertakes a careful examination of the neck and that the cervical spine is put through a full range of active and passive movement to try and determine the precise level and extent of the lesion. It may be necessary to hold each spinal position for 10 to 15 seconds to reproduce symptoms. A hurried examination must not be carried out.

Investigations

Plain radiographs including obliques, although useful, must be interpreted with caution. A myelogram or vertebral angiogram may rarely be needed for more precise localisation of the lesion. Other investigations such as erythrocyte sedimentation rates and examination of the cerebrospinal fluid will not help except in excluding other diseases. Nerve conduction studies and electromyography may help to decide which nerve roots are involved.

Treatment

Acute symptoms, which are very painful, require rest for the neck and strong analgesics, even opiates (Chapter 15). A collar or neck traction is usually required and in most patients will lead to a resolution of symptoms. Very rarely surgical decompression will be necessary. Occasionally in such cases, myelography may be followed by a deterioration in the patient's condition and such investigations should not be undertaken unless operating theatre facilities are available.

Characteristically chronic symptoms tend to come and go and require the use of mild analgesics, a restriction in activity, attention to neck posture and usually the use of a cervical collar. Many patients, either on their own or their doctor's advice become martyrs to the use of a collar. In general, the majority of patients will do well with the intermittent use of a soft felt, Sorbo-rubber or Plastazote collar at night. This should be used in conjunction with a single soft pillow. Such management relieves the early morning symptoms of which most patients complain, sets the patient up well for the day ahead and avoids the cosmetic problems of wearing a collar during the day. Patients may need encouragement and even a sedative to acquire this collar-wearing habit. A small proportion of patients will require the use of firmer collars by day and night. It is important that such collars are made in a position of comfort, usually in slight flexion, and that localised pressure areas do not develop.

In this group of patients a programme of neck traction may be useful, once the optimum position for relief of pain has been found. Modest weights (up to 5kg or 10lb) are usually employed although some advocate much larger weights. Great care must be taken with traction in patients with unstable necks and in those with rheumatoid arthritis, and very small weights should be used.

Spinal manipulation has its advocates. Such treatment is potentially dangerous in inexperienced hands, particularly in the presence of an acute lesion. (See Chapter 14.)

Caution should be used in interpreting the results of the above-mentioned treatment, or indeed of persisting unduly with time-consuming programmes of treatment, as studies show that most patients improve within three months whatever treatment is given.

In some cases surgical fusion of adjacent vertebrae may be required or rarely decompression. Such treatment is often technically difficult and may lead to increased demands (and the possibility of increased symptoms) upon the remainder of the spine.

Muscle and ligamentous symptoms will respond to simple analgesics, accurate local injections of anaesthetic and corticosteroids, to relaxing measures such as heat, and muscle-relaxing drugs (e.g. Valium) and to simple exercise programmes. Indeed, when symptoms from whatever cause have been relieved, a suitable exercise programme should strengthen muscles and this will afford a protective influence.

Symptoms due to vertebral artery compression are helped by reducing neck movements by the use of a collar, although neck traction and exercise programmes must be avoided. Surgical decompression of the vessel may be required.

DIFFERENTIAL DIAGNOSIS OF CERVICAL SPINAL DISEASE

Acute disc lesions, particularly if due to trauma, may be confused with vertebral fracture or compression. The symptoms of chronic disc protrusion associated with cord compression must be distinguished from multiple sclerosis, cord tumours, motor neurone disease, syringomyelia and sub-acute degeneration of the cord due to Vitamin B_{12} deficiency.

The spinal apophyseal joints may be involved in a variety of inflammatory diseases which will require anti-inflammatory drugs (Chapter 15). Such diseases include rheumatoid arthritis, ankylosing spondylitis, psoriatic arthritis and Reiter's disease (Chapter 7). A variety of cardiovascular diseases may impair vertebral artery blood flow including atherosclerosis, cardiac valvular disease, thrombosis and embolism.

Spinal tumour or infective lesions (tuberculosis, staphylococcus, etc.) may cause nerve root symptoms. Herpes zoster (shingles) may cause similar nerve root symptoms and diagnostic confusion until the typical vesicular rash appears. Involvement of more than one or two nerve roots suggests damage to the brachial plexus, as with viral radiculitis, thoracic outlet syndromes and drooping of the shoulders with marked downward movement of the outer end of the clavicle, often found in middle-aged women.

DORSAL SPINE

Although dorsal spinal abnormalities are found commonly in radiographic studies of the general population, the incidence of symptoms is low. Nerve root symptoms are the commonest with pain radiating to the front of the chest or abdomen. The pain may simulate that arising from thoracic or abdominal viscera.

Treatment may include use of analgesics, a firm bed, extension and rotation exercises, weight reduction, the use of a firm brassière for those with heavy or pendulous breasts, a full posterior spinal support, and occasionally nerve root blocks.

LUMBAR SPINE

Clinical Features

There are some differences between the type and causes of symptoms in the lumbar spine compared with the cervical spine. In particular, there are no vascular symptoms. Ninety per cent of symptoms affect the L5 or S1 roots. The symptoms in order of frequency are:

a) Symptoms due to trauma or degenerative changes in the intervertebral discs or spinal joints producing pain and muscle spasm in the associated spinal dermatome (see Plate 11/6 and Fig. 11/2).

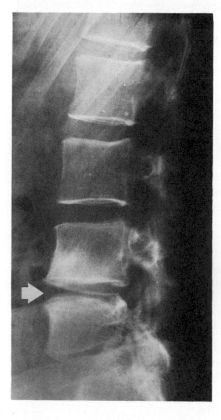

Plate 11/6 A lateral radiograph of the lumbar spine showing degenerative changes with narrowing of the L4-5 disc and loss of the lumbar curve due to protective muscle spasm

b) Symptoms due to damage in muscles and ligaments produced by trauma, abnormal loading or bad posture. If close to the skin surface the signs may be localised but are usually similar to (a).

c) Symptoms due to pressure of osteophytes or postero-lateral disc protrusion on the spinal nerves.

d) Symptoms due to pressure of osteophytes or central disc protrusion on the cauda equina. The spinal cord terminates at the level of the second lumbar vertebra.

The use of the standard examination technique which is listed in Table 1, will ensure that nothing is omitted.

SYMPTOMS (A) AND (B)

Changes which fall short of actual nerve compression cause local pain
and produce an area of referred pain, often called lumbago, which is
listed in Table II. The pain is deep-seated and nagging, and may be
associated with muscle spasm and reduced spinal motion.

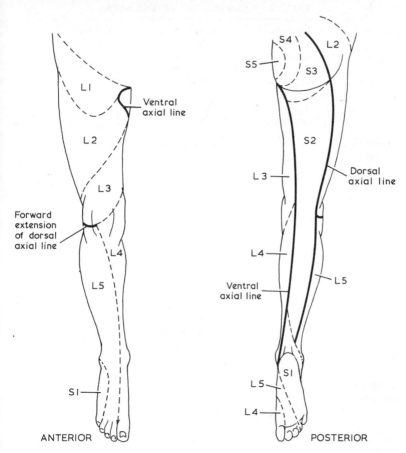

Fig. 11/2 Plan of the dermatomes of the lower limb

SYMPTOMS (C)

Nerve compression produces similar or more severe pain but in
addition there are motor effects which are listed in Table II and
altered, reduced or absent sensation in the areas shown in Fig. 11/2.

Plantar and dorsiflexors are best tested with the foot on the ground with the patient standing or sitting respectively. There is muscle spasm, often with reduction in lumbar lordosis and mild lumbar scoliosis. It must be appreciated that there are individual variations in nerve distribution and the listed effects must be interpreted with caution.

TABLE I   EXAMINATION OF THE BACK

Position	Musculo-skeletal system	Central nervous system	Referred pain
Standing	Inspection Range of back movement	Plantar flexor power	
Kneeling Sitting		Ankle reflex Dorsiflexor power	
Bending over table Sitting on table	Palpation	Knee reflex	
Lying supine	Range of hip movement	Straight leg raising Quadriceps and hamstring power Sensation on front of leg Plantar reflex	Abdominal examination
Lying on left side		Right hip abductor power	
Lying on right side		Left hip abductor power	
Lying prone		Femoral stretch test Gluteus maximus tone Saddle anaesthesia	Rectal examination

TABLE II   LUMBAR NERVE ROOT SYMPTOMS AND SIGNS

Spinal segment and root involved	Area of referred deep pain	Muscle weakness and wasting	Reduced or absent reflexes
L2	Upper buttock, groin	Hip flexors, adductors	
L3	Mid-buttock, anterior aspect of thigh	Hip flexors, adductors Quadriceps	Knee
L4	Lower buttock, round lateral aspect of thigh to anterior aspect of knee	Quadriceps Tibialis anterior	Knee
L5	Lower buttock, lateral aspect of thigh and calf	Tibialis posterior Peronei Toe extensors	Ankle
S1	Posterior aspect of thigh and calf	Calf and toe flexors Hamstrings, glutei	Ankle

Nerve compression is associated with nerve irritation detected by reduced straight leg raising with a positive Lasègue's sign or hip extension with the knee flexed (sciatic and femoral nerve stretch tests). Nerve compression symptoms in the distribution of the sciatic nerve, constitute sciatica, a term often abused by medical and lay people. The symptoms from a prolapsed disc are usually aggravated by straightening up from a stooping position far more than bending, lifting weights, coughing, sneezing and straining at defaecation. The pain is eased by rest, each patient having a preferred position.

SYMPTOMS (D)

Cauda equina compression is a most serious condition. Involvement of all the nerves may occur with profound motor and sensory changes in the legs. Saddle anaesthesia and absence of buttock muscle tone are signs of S3 to 5 root damage. Further, involvement of the sacral nerves will produce additional motor and sensory changes but, more importantly, sphincter disturbances with retention of urine and faeces. Similar cauda equina symptoms may appear slowly with a spinal tumour or with spinal stenosis. In spinal stenosis, which is due to developmental or bony changes reducing the space available for the spinal cord, the compression symptoms may be exercise-related and may improve with rest, suggesting a vascular component to the symptoms which is not present.

Involvement of individual spinal joints, ligaments and muscles in inflammatory or traumatic processes will give rise to muscle spasm and pain in the distributions listed in Table II.

INVESTIGATION AND TREATMENT OF LUMBAR SPINE LESIONS

The physiotherapist must assess the lumbar spine in the manner described for the cervical spine. However, in the lumbar spine, psychological factors are probably more important as almost everyone has had backache at some time, and most people feel that backache is an inevitable result of the stresses of modern living. Backache is a major cause of loss of work but not all cases have significant pathological lesions in their spines. In other cases the backache may be related to an injury for which the patient is claiming compensation and in most cases this will complicate assessment. In many of these patients symptoms will not finally clear until adequate compensation has been received, usually three to four years later.

Investigations

Plain radiographs must be interpreted with caution as changes in the lumbar spine are very common with increasing age and bear little relation to symptoms. Oblique rather than lateral radiographs are required to demonstrate the apophyseal joints. A myelogram may be required to localise both root and cauda equina lesions (Plates 11/7 and 8). Examination of the cerebrospinal fluid and other investigations are of little value except in excluding other conditions (Table

Plate 11/7 (*below*) A myelogram showing a disc protrusion at the level of L4–5 with a less marked protrusion at the L3–4 level

Plate 11/8 (*right*) A myelogram showing spinal stenosis with failure of the dye to extend below the middle of the fourth lumbar vertebra. The spinal stenosis is due to extensive degenerative changes which are clearly visible

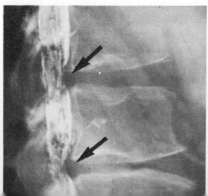
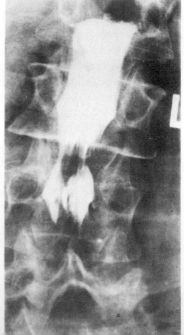

III). In some cases nerve conduction studies and electromyography may help to decide which nerves and muscles are involved.

Treatment

Most patients experience relief of pain with clearing of the neurological symptoms and signs if a basic programme of treatment is followed.

DRUGS

The use of full dosage of a simple analgesic often supplemented by a muscle relaxant such as Valium. In severe cases opiates may be required.

REST

Ideally the patient should have complete bed rest, with no pillows, on a firm mattress supported by boards for a period of up to three weeks. After an acute attack, patients should be encouraged to persist with such arrangements for sleeping each night; if necessary for ever. Most patients prefer a firm bed, once they have tried it.

In most patients it is unnecessary to proceed further, since symptoms will settle after a few days of this treatment.

TRACTION

For patients who do not settle quickly with rest, light traction may be required. Although 1·5–2kg (3–4lb) is usually sufficient, some recommend much heavier traction.

MANIPULATION

Some advocate spinal manipulation. Such treatment, when undertaken by properly trained experts, is often beneficial and in sequential radiographs has been shown to reduce disc protrusion. In the face of massive central disc protrusion such manipulation can be very dangerous. Patients must be X-rayed before manipulation and it should be avoided if there is substantial root pain, bilateral root pain, possible bladder involvement, severe osteoporosis or inflammatory joint disease.

SPINAL SUPPORTS

For those patients who cannot afford the time for bed rest, a plaster jacket may produce the same results in an acute attack. It needs to be worn for at least four weeks and often for longer. Symptoms which are unchanged after two to four weeks in such a jacket must be re-assessed carefully. Such treatment should reduce the symptoms and failure to do so suggests other causes or perhaps psychological factors. In the recovery phase use of some spinal support, preferably a properly made surgical corset, is important. Many patients require to use such support intermittently over many years.

PHYSIOTHERAPY

Patients may find simple local heating a useful adjunct to an exercise programme as muscle spasm and pain will be reduced. Patients need to be taught a simple regime of spinal exercises that they can carry out not only for a few weeks while symptoms persist but also for many years in an attempt to reduce the relapse rate. At the same time patients must be taught how to lift, and to be conscious of their posture at all times.

WEIGHT REDUCTION

This may be vital if repeated attacks are to be avoided, and the physiotherapist can do much to reinforce this information.

SURGERY

Surgical decompression must be undertaken quickly in patients with cauda equina compression. This will require laminectomy and removal of the prolapsed material. In those with more chronic symptoms due to disc protrusion or osteophytes, unresponsive to other treatment, surgical removal of the compressing material may be required. In patients with very persistent symptoms, particularly if these are arising from the apophyseal joints, spinal fusion may be required. Some surgeons recommend spinal fusion as a primary procedure at the time of removal of the prolapsed material. However, these major operations must only be undertaken after careful assessment of the patient, as a disturbing number of patients continue to have symptoms despite apparently successful surgical treatment.

DIFFERENTIAL DIAGNOSIS OF BACKACHE

Although the conditions described above are the commonest causes of backache, the complaint is so frequently encountered in the general practitioner's surgery and in the orthopaedic clinic that other conditions must be remembered. It is easy for both patients and medical personnel to dismiss low backache as an inevitable consequence of the human race having adopted an upright posture. Table III lists some of the conditions which may cause low backache.

Vertebral fracture due to trauma, osteoporosis or neoplastic deposit is the only common cause of acute symptoms apart from acute disc

TABLE III   COMMONER CAUSES OF LOW BACKACHE

Cause		Investigations	
		Radiological	Other
Congenital	Short leg		
	Sacralised L5	Diagnosis	
	Lumbarised S1	,,	
	Spondylolysis	,,	
	Spondylolisthesis	,,	
Traumatic	Prolapsed disc	Myelogram	
	Ligamentous tear		
	Fracture	Diagnosis	
Degenerative	Osteoarthrosis	Diagnosis	
	Hyperostosis	,,	
Inflammatory	Ankylosing spondylitis	Sacro-iliitis	ESR
	Reiter's disease	,,	,,
	Colitic arthritis	,,	,,
	Psoriatic arthritis	,,	,,
	Pyogenic osteomyelitis	Helpful	,, , white cell count
	Tuberculosis	,,	,, , white cell count
	Osteochondritis	Diagnosis	
Neoplastic	Secondary deposit	Helpful	Bone scan, Alkaline phosphatase
	Myeloma	,,	ESR, bone marrow
	Spinal cord tumour	Myelogram	
	Primary bone tumour	Helpful	Bone scan, Alkaline phosphatase
Metabolic	Osteoporosis	Changes	Calcium, phosphorus,
	Osteomalacia	often Diagnostic	Alkaline phosphatase
	Paget's disease	Diagnosis	Alkaline phosphatase
	Pyrophosphate arthritis	,,	
Postural	Pregnancy		
	Obesity		
	Occupational		
	Hip disease	Diagnosis	
	Scoliosis	,,	
Other system disease	Gynaecological		
	Renal	IVP	Local examination
	Rectal	Barium enema	

protrusion and muscle or ligamentous tears. Further, there are age-related diseases in that osteochondritis (Scheuermann's disease) affects those under 15 years and neoplastic disease, osteoporosis and Paget's disease are uncommon in those under 50 years.

Assessment of low backache requires a full examination of the spine with the patient undressed, examination of the sacro-iliac and hip joints, measurement of leg length, a neurological examination and sufficient general examination to exclude the possibility of tumour (myeloma and secondary deposits from primary tumours in the lung, breast, kidney, prostate and thyroid glands are the commonest). Bowel and gynaecological diseases may cause backache and appropriate examination including rectal and vaginal examination will be required. The minimum radiographic requirements are an antero-posterior view of the lumbar spine and pelvis, a lateral view of the lumbar spine and a coned view of the lumbo-sacral junction. All patients over the age of 40 years should have a chest radiograph. The other relevant tests are shown in Table III.

BIBLIOGRAPHY

See end of Chapter 12.

Chapter 12

Orthopaedic Surgical Procedures

by A. G. MOWAT, m.b., f.r.c.p. (Ed.) and C. P. ROBERTS, m.c.s.p.

Surgical procedures are being increasingly used at all stages of joint disease, particularly in rheumatoid arthritis. In this disease approximately 10 per cent of patients attending out-patient clinics would benefit from an orthopaedic procedure although for a variety of reasons it may not be possible to carry out all the operations deemed beneficial. In osteoarthrosis the patient load is even greater. The steady advance in prosthetic surgery, particularly for the hip joint, has led to an increased demand for surgical treatment of osteoarthrosis and in many areas there is a two or more year waiting list. The true demand may be even higher based upon surveys of the disabled in the community but with waiting lists of this duration many patients are simply not referred to hospital departments unless the disability and pain are severe. Since there is no immediate prospect of increasing the cold orthopaedic surgical service it is especially important that careful selection of the patients who are likely to gain the most benefit is undertaken and, along with others in the management team, the physiotherapist has an important part to play in such patient selection.

Although patients with inflammatory disease, especially rheumatoid arthritis, clearly have different disease characteristics and requirements compared with patients with osteoarthrosis, the same general principles of assessment and treatment apply. However, it is helpful if the major differences which are described in other chapters are listed.

INFLAMMATORY JOINT DISEASE

1. Younger patients
2. Requirements reflect their age. Employment and sexual aspects may be important

3. Multiple joint disease influences the results and makes the return to normal function unlikely
4. Systemic features, particularly widespread muscle wasting, will limit the functional improvement

OSTEOARTHROSIS

1. Old patients
2. Requirements reflect their age. Normal domestic and social activities and retirement pleasures are their aims
3. The disease predominantly affects a single joint making a 'cure' with a full return of function possible
4. Cardio-pulmonary problems may cause operative difficulties but rarely influence the functional results

This chapter will include aspects of patient selection applicable to both diseases, highlight possible pre-, per- and postoperative problems and indicate the types of operative treatment available. This chapter will *not* include a description of the detailed physiotherapeutic regimes used for each surgical operation as it is assumed that the therapist is familiar with the basic principles of, and the methods employed in, the development of muscle strength and control. This chapter only includes details of patient management where these have been found to be valuable or important. Further, such management must be considered against a background of total management as described in other chapters. It must also be appreciated that many orthopaedic surgeons advocate highly individualised programmes of management and that the programmes described in this chapter are not necessarily the only, or the 'correct' forms of management. They have, however, been shown to be effective.

AIMS OF SURGICAL TREATMENT

The aims of surgical treatment are three-fold.

1. *An improvement in function.* Such improvement may relate to the domestic, social, economic, employment or sexual implications of the patient's deformity and disability. In essence almost all treatment is directed towards an improvement in function, since it is functional difficulties of which the patients complain.

2. *Relief of pain.* Many surgeons will argue that relief of pain is the prime and often the only reason for operation. Such an approach may imply the inability of the operation or prosthesis to improve function, but more usually reflects greater difficulty in demonstrating improved

postoperative function than pain relief. In most cases pain relief leads to a functional improvement. However, in some instances surgical treatment may not improve function, particularly when a joint is arthrodesed, but may simply allow the patient to sit or sleep without pain.

3. *Improvement in appearance.* In most patients the deterioration in function and appearance will have taken place gradually and they are much more concerned about function than appearance. Thus it is uncommon, except in young women, and some patients with juvenile chronic polyarthritis, to operate for cosmetic reasons alone. However, it must be admitted that an improvement in appearance can be a great morale booster.

PATIENT ASSESSMENT

In osteoarthrosis the surgical decision is simply whether to operate, while in rheumatoid arthritis the surgical decisions of whether to operate and if so upon which joint, are often difficult to make. This is partly due to the complex disabilities arising from multiple joint disease and partly because almost all orthopaedic surgery, in contrast to most other surgical treatments, is both elective and demanding upon the patient. Thus, except in the case of stabilisation of the upper cervical spine, the surgery has little or no effect upon the patient's general health or life expectancy. Further, many procedures place considerable demands upon the patient, particularly in co-operating fully with the physiotherapist, if a satisfactory result is to be achieved.

A correct surgical decision will usually be made if all members of the arthritis team can independently assess the patient's difficulties and likely response to treatment and then arrive at a conference decision, on whether to operate and upon which joint. It will be obvious from the following discussion the information and advice that is expected from the physiotherapist. The final decisions on the type of operation must then be made by the surgeon and physician in the light of various technical and medical considerations discussed later. Such assessment should concentrate upon the following factors.

The Patient's Requirements

The patient's requirements must be clearly identified. These will, as suggested above, usually be centred upon an improvement in function. To this end the paramedical and nursing staff should undertake, as far as possible, a practical measurement of the patient's domestic, social, employment and sexual difficulties. For example, it is easy to accept as reasonable a patient's wish to be able to walk to the shops when a home visit will quickly show that none of the therapeutic alternatives could possibly provide the required functional improvement.

Local Joint Disease

Measurement of existing muscle strength, joint movement and stability together with radiographs, will allow an assessment of how these might be influenced by exercises and surgery.

Extent and Severity of the Arthritis

An evaluation of the arthritis is vital since response to surgery will be influenced by involvement of other joints. Thus the results of knee surgery may be affected not only by hip and foot involvement but also by the patient's ability to use carefully selected walking aids with his upper limbs in the immediate postoperative period. Further, experience shows that in patients requiring both hip and knee surgery, the hip operation should be undertaken first as this facilitates subsequent mobilisation of the knees; and stabilisation and relief of pain at the wrist may make subsequent hand surgery unnecessary.

The Patient's Mental Response

The patient's mental response to her disease and disability must be assessed and hence judgement made upon her likely co-operation in achieving satisfactory postoperative progress and the optimum result. Patients are naturally anxious to appear to conform to normal patterns of behaviour and can be expected to claim that a return towards previous functional levels is their major wish. However detailed and unhurried assessment and examination of the response to earlier therapeutic efforts and hospitalisation may show that they really do not wish or require a major change in function or that they cannot co-operate in an extended and physically and mentally demanding period of treatment away from home.

Family Response

An assessment must be made after interview, and ideally a home visit, of the reaction of the patient's family to the disease. In many families, patterns of activity and responsibility will have evolved over the years and will have become both convenient and fixed, so that improved function may not be utilised. Further, a first hand view of the domestic architecture may show that despite its capacity for simple adaptation the demands placed upon the patient will remain too great and the results of the contemplated surgery will never be utilised.

It is fashionable to talk of patient motivation and to ascribe success or failure to the patient's good or bad motivation. It should now be clear that with proper pre-operative assessment little should be left to chance in arriving at the correct surgical decision.

GENERAL SURGICAL CONSIDERATIONS

The Patient's General Health

As with any elective operation the patient's cardio-respiratory reserve must be adequate. Patients with osteoarthrosis who are anaemic may require appropriate investigation and the treatment of the anaemia pre-operatively. However, many patients with rheumatoid arthritis are anaemic, the anaemia being proportional to the activity of the disease, and there is no evidence to show that there is an increased risk in operating upon patients who have adapted to haemoglobin values as low as 10·5g/dl. Those with lower values are best transfused a few days pre-operatively.

It is often supposed that surgical wounds are more liable to become infected and to heal poorly in rheumatoid patients compared with osteoarthrotic patients and it is further supposed that treatment with corticosteroids is likely to exaggerate these tendencies. However, in practice there is no difference in wound healing in the two patient groups and it is unnecessary to impose a reduced rate of postoperative mobilisation or delay in stitch removal in patients with rheumatoid arthritis.

Although analgesic drugs can be withdrawn in patients with osteoarthrosis, in rheumatoid arthritis all drug therapy should be continued over the operative period lest there be an increase in general disease symptoms. It is common practice to perhaps double the dose of any corticosteroid drug for 24 to 48 hours using intramuscular injections of hydrocortisone. However this is probably both unnecessary and unwise. The plasma cortisol value rises rapidly during surgical procedures while additional corticosteroid therapy may be associated with an increased risk of wound or intercurrent infection.

Major hip and knee surgery is associated with an increased incidence of deep venous thrombosis and pulmonary embolism and many orthopaedic surgeons employ some form of anti-coagulation. Although this subject is still open to debate, the current view is that patients with osteoarthrosis undergoing these procedures should be anti-coagulated with warfarin, while for reasons that are not fully understood, such anti-coagulation is generally unnecessary in patients with rheumatoid arthritis. However, anti-coagulation in both patient groups is mandatory if there is a history of previous thrombo-embolic disease.

The Patient's Local Disease

Although it is important that the patient should be receiving any necessary drugs or physical therapy in an attempt to reduce the inflammatory reaction, it is unnecessary to control the activity of the local joint disease before operating. However, procedures involving synovectomy may be simpler if the synovial inflammation is controlled and the vascularity of the tissue reduced by a short period of rest. In particular it is an advantage to correct deformities secondary to inflammation, such as flexion of the knee, since such correction will simplify the surgical procedure and the resultant improvement in muscle control and development will speed postoperative recovery.

Patient Handling and Intubation

The anaesthetist and all who handle the cervical spine of the unconscious rheumatoid patient must remember that many have an unstable neck (see Chapter 6). Since the majority of patients are symptomless and radiographs are unhelpful in predicting those that are likely to have trouble, all must be handled carefully. We send every patient to the operating theatre in a soft collar, which although it is removed, serves as a useful reminder to the theatre staff.

Occasionally involvement of the temporo-mandibular joint will limit mouth opening, while in a few patients, usually those with juvenile chronic polyarthritis which has extended into adult life, the cervical spine may have ankylosed, presenting even greater difficulties with intubation. Patients with ankylosing spondylitis may have the same problem.

TECHNICAL CONSIDERATIONS

Finally, when the decision to operate has been reached the surgeon must consider a number of technical factors. Clearly better results are achieved when the surgeon is familiar with the particular procedure to be used. In consequence, most surgeons have a limited repertoire of operations and only change to a new technique when it has been shown to have definite advantages over that currently employed. To this end, it is important that periodic reviews of a Unit's overall operative results are undertaken; it is all too easy to gain false impressions by seeing patients occasionally in busy follow-up clinics. Since it is impossible with surgical operations to imitate the double-blind method used in the assessment of drug and physical therapy, it is important that the review is undertaken by an independent assessor.

The range of movement available with some operations may be greater than with others but may be achieved with some reduction in stability. In general, excision arthroplasty leads to less stability than prosthetic arthroplasty and this is particularly the case in the hip and elbow. Such considerations may also be important if it becomes necessary to remove an infected prosthesis leaving a joint with a good range of movement but considerable instability.

The use of a tourniquet imposes restrictions on the time available for operations distal to the shoulder and hip joints. The operative time is restricted to approximately one and a half hours with further restrictions if the patient has significant peripheral arteriosclerosis or vasculitis.

Patients with rheumatoid arthritis often have perceptible thinning of the skin, with some loss of subcutaneous fat and connective tissues supporting blood vessels. These changes can lead to marked bruising of the limbs, occasionally associated with shearing and subsequent loss of an area of skin, during manipulation of a limb to facilitate insertion of a prosthesis. The most vulnerable area is over the shin. Additional care and the pre-operative application of foam or other protective bandages to the limbs will reduce these problems.

Infection of a Prosthetic Joint

Several studies have shown that patients with rheumatoid arthritis have a higher incidence of prosthetic infection than do patients with osteoarthrosis; the incidence is greater in both groups if the joint has been the site of a previous operation, whether or not a prosthesis was employed. While there is still debate over the need for special operating theatres for prosthetic surgery, the possibility of infection of a prosthesis from a septic focus elsewhere in the body must always be considered, as it constitutes a major surgical disaster.

Although it is debated whether prostheses, particularly metallic prostheses, whether fixed with bone cement or not, have a special tendency to attract bacterial organisms, undoubtedly there is a risk of infection of a prosthesis if it is inserted while the patient has a bacteraemia. There is growing evidence that late infection is due to blood spread rather than being a manifestation of infection at the time of surgery. It follows that septic foci in nails and rheumatoid nodules should be eradicated and any infection of the urinary tract or chest treated energetically, not only pre-operatively but whenever they occur in a patient with a metal implant. Dental sepsis, more likely in the younger rheumatoid patients than the older osteoarthrotic patient with dentures, also needs to be considered. Finally, the high incidence of foot sepsis in patients with rheumatoid arthritis presents a special risk to lower limb prostheses and emphasises the value of correcting foot problems by the provision of suitable footwear or surgical treatment before hips or knees are subjected to prosthetic surgery.

TYPES OF OPERATION

There are four major types of operation currently used in the joints of patients with arthrosis – synovectomy/debridement, arthroplasty, osteotomy and arthrodesis.

Synovectomy/Debridement

In osteoarthrosis loose bodies or osteophytes which are causing joint locking or impeding normal joint motion may be removed, the operation usually being performed on the knee or elbow joints. Meniscectomy can be regarded as a similar type of operation.

Synovectomy is undertaken in inflammatory arthritis. The chief indications are pain and swelling of the joint unresponsive to medical therapy. At present the operation is considered of some value when performed on finger joints, the wrist, elbow and knee joint. Although encouraging results of synovectomy have been reported in damaged joints, most stress that the operation must be performed early, usually after three to six months of persistent disease, before significant cartilage and bone damage have occurred, to obtain the best results. Early uncontrolled studies tended to support the hope that the operation would have a prophylactic effect and that the rate of joint damage would at least be retarded if not halted. However, it has become clear that this was a forlorn hope. It must be emphasised that synovectomy produces reasonably predictable results in terms of relief of pain and swelling for periods of three to five years. Follow-up studies indicate a steady deterioration in the percentage of good results from up to 80 per cent at one year to 50 per cent or less at five years. However, since the operation is associated with all the usual surgical risks, may lead to significant loss of movement particularly in finger joints, requires in-patient treatment for approximately three weeks in the case of a knee joint, and has now been shown not to have a prophylactic value, its place in management is being questioned. Since similar results are claimed for radio-isotope injections a number of workers are optimistic that this form of treatment may partly replace synovectomy, particularly as it requires only two or three days in hospital and is associated with fewer short term problems.

Synovectomy of tendon sheaths, particularly those of the fingers, remains a valuable procedure. The operation relieves pain and improves tendon function and in some cases may be urgently required to protect the extensor tendons of the fingers from stretching or rupture. This operation does appear to be prophylactic and the long term results remain very satisfactory.

Arthroplasty

Any operation which reconstitutes the joint is described as an arthroplasty. In a few cases the operation consists simply of excision of the damaged joint surfaces and synovial tissue, e.g. metacarpophalangeal joints, metatarsophalangeal joints, lower end of ulna, elbow and hip. However, with the success of total hip replacement prostheses are being increasingly used to replace part or the whole of the joint.

Osteotomy

Division of a bone near to a joint, but outside the joint capsule, has been a useful and popular operation for treatment of osteoarthrosis particularly in the hip and knee. The operation allows weight to be carried through a different, largely undamaged portion of the articular cartilage and in addition may also reduce pain, particularly night pain, by inducing changes in venous blood flow. There is good evidence that the procedure encourages the coverage of denuded areas of bone by fibrocartilage. However, in patients with rheumatoid arthritis it is usual to find the whole joint cartilage affected by the inflammatory process and therefore changes in the load bearing have little application.

Arthrodesis

The pathological process in rheumatoid arthritis may lead to fibrous and occasionally bony ankylosis, particularly at the wrist. Since such ankylosis usually produces an improvement in function, there has long been a surgical tradition of arthrodesing peripheral joints to produce the same effect. Undoubtedly there are good clinical indications for arthrodesing such joints as the wrist, elbow, knee, ankle and sub-talar joints, provided the correct position for arthrodesis and the possible difficulties for the patient have been adequately assessed and explained beforehand. Arthrodesis of these joints should not be dismissed as outdated in the face of the current obsession with the retention of movement.

SURGICAL PROCEDURES FOR INDIVIDUAL JOINTS

Forefeet

The first metatarsal phalangeal joint in patients with osteoarthrosis frequently requires surgical treatment. Hallux rigidus may be treated by arthrodesis or excision arthroplasty while hallux valgus is usually treated by Keller's arthroplasty; excision of part of the proximal phalanx and the toe position maintained by insertion of K-wires across the joint for two to three weeks. Walking training in protective plaster or bandages can be commenced as soon as postoperative swelling has settled, usually after three to five days.

In rheumatoid arthritis a combination of initial inflammatory changes and secondary mechanical factors at the metatarsophalangeal joints produces the characteristic broadening and rigidity of the forefoot with hallux valgus, deviation of the other toes in a lateral direction, subluxation of the toes on to the dorsum of the foot, and the development of callosities over the prominent metatarsal heads in the

Plate 12/1 The typical deformities of feet with rheumatoid arthritis

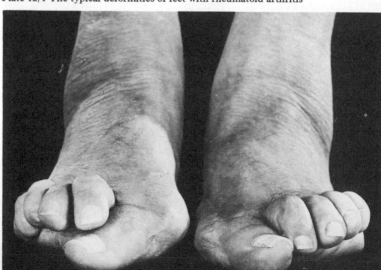

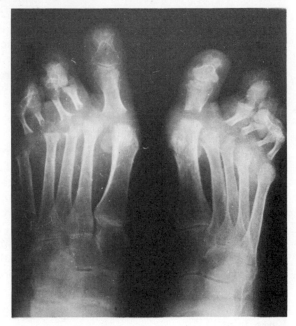

Plate 12/2
Radiograph of the feet showing bilateral excision arthroplasties of the metatarsal phalangeal joints

sole (Plate 12/1). The normal protective fibro-fatty pad is drawn forward off the metatarsal heads and the callosities develop in an attempt to protect the inflamed and tender tissues. Early symptoms should be treated conservatively as synovectomy has little to offer. However, as the disease progresses and if conservative therapy in the form of suitable domed insoles, changes in shoes, the use of metatarsal bars and the provision of custom-made shoes fails, excision arthroplasty for the metatarsophalangeal joints should be considered. The results of this procedure are so satisfactory that there is no place for joint replacement.

Excision arthroplasty with removal of the metatarsal heads and/or the bases of the proximal phalanges and manipulation of the toes into normal alignment produces satisfactory results in 90 per cent of cases (Plate 12/2). Poor results are due to insufficient or irregular excision of bone. Grossly deformed toes may be amputated. Swelling may occur following foot surgery, with some impairment in wound healing and consequently a delay in walking. Different surgical groups favour early removal of the pressure bandage, the use of Buerger's exercises to reduce oedema, early ambulation from the second or third day, or the use of various forms of custom-made shoes to control the distribution of weight and to speed healing and consequently the patient's discharge from hospital. In general it is best to operate on both feet at the same time even though one may show relatively minor damage, since the patient's greatest functional gain is the ability to wear a normal pair of shoes. However if only one foot is operated upon, advice as to where the patient can find shops that are willing to sell odd size shoes will be much appreciated.

Mid-Tarsal, Sub-Talar and Ankle Joints

Involvement of these joints is best treated by provision of suitable shoes or boots with valgus insoles, various forms of anklet, plastic heel cups and even a leg iron and T-strap may adequately support these joints. Occasionally, simple manipulation under anaesthesia followed by ice treatment and exercises reduces pain and restores movement.

Arthrodesis is the most satisfactory operation. The ankle should be fused in 5° of plantar flexion in men and 10° in women with the foot and heel fixed in neutral positions. Although prostheses for the ankle joint exist, experience is as yet limited and indications for their use are not clearly defined.

Knee Joint

Principal movements at the knee are flexion and extension but antero-posterior glide, abduction, adduction and rotation are all possible, the last being particularly important for normal knee function. Owing to the shape of the femoral condyles flexion and extension occur round a continuously changing axis. Movement of the knee is further complicated by the presence of the menisci which are important in joint lubrication, have a shock absorbing role and between them carry up to 7 per cent of the load transmitted across the joint. Finally, the patella contributes to full and normal function of the quadriceps mechanism.

There have been several consequences of a better understanding of the mechanics of the knee joint.

1. There has been a reluctance to remove menisci unless they are frankly torn or severely damaged.

2. There has also been a reluctance to undertake patellectomy, either alone or as part of an arthroplasty, since postoperative progress and restoration of quadriceps strength is slower.

3. There has been a marked swing away from linked rigidly bone-fixed hinge prostheses towards non-linked, carefully designed prostheses which maintain the changing centre of axis of movement during flexion and extension and which allow the final 'screw-home' rotation

of the femur medially on the tibia as the knee approaches full extension.

SYNOVECTOMY

In patients with rheumatoid arthritis synovectomy of the knee joint remains a useful procedure for relief of pain and swelling and recurrent effusion. As indicated earlier the possible prophylactic benefits of the procedure have not been realised and there is now a less pressing demand for early surgical treatment in a joint unresponsive to conservative therapy. Anterior synovectomy is usually performed and may also be valuable in those with an enlarged posterior cyst (Plate 12/3). Such cysts, which are usually extensions of the normal semimembranosus-gastrocnemius bursae may become grossly enlarged, prevent full knee extension and cause venous obstruction. In addition, since they are connected to the knee joint by a one-way valvular mechanism, they are subject to markedly increased fluid pressures. This may result in the enlargement of the cyst into the calf or the sudden rupture of the cyst with the release of irritant synovial fluid (Plate 12/4). Symptoms and signs of joint rupture, which have also been recorded at the wrist and elbow, mimic those of a deep venous thrombosis. Arthrography should be used to establish the diagnosis. Rupture of the cyst should be treated by rest. A large calf cyst may be excised but synovectomy of the joint treats the cause of both a small cyst and rupture.

Plate 12/3 An arthrogram – lateral view of the right knee – showing a proliferated synovial lining in the joint and a large posterior cyst extending down the calf

Plate 12/4 An arthrogram – medial view of the right knee – showing rupture of the joint with leakage of the dye into the calf. Note that the appearance is not cystic and the margins are not distinct

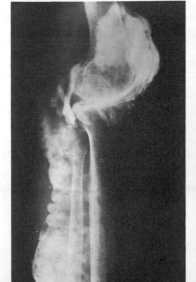
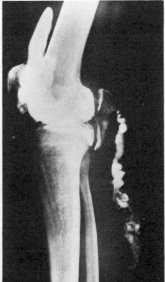

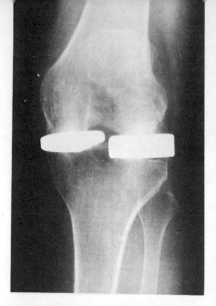

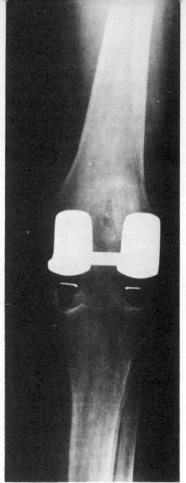

Plate 12/5 (*above*) Radiograph showing bi-compartmental MacIntosh arthroplasties in a rheumatoid knee. Prostheses of different depth allow replacement of damaged tibial surfaces, correction of the deformity and restoration of joint stability

Plate 12/6 (*right*) Radiograph of a Geomedic total knee replacement. The femoral replacement is metal while the tibial replacement is of polyethylene and only the marker wires show on the radiograph

ARTHROPLASTY

Despite the suggestions of some surgeons that inter-position arthroplasty, of which the MacIntosh tibial replacement is an example, is only of historical interest, many still feel that until the new total replacement prostheses have been shown to have long-term success there remain clear indications for this type of operation (Plate 12/5). The indications include a moderately damaged joint with only minimal damage to the femoral condyle, since in essence the condyle continues to articulate with the replaced tibial condyle, and a range of flexion of 80° since movement is rarely improved by this operation; while a valgus or varus deformity of 20° and a flexion deformity of 20° can both be corrected by the operation. Synovectomy is undertaken at the same time while only a thin sliver of bone is removed from the tibial plateau. The range of prostheses of different depth and length allow angular deformity to be corrected and ligamentous stability to be improved.

Total replacement arthroplasty is being increasingly employed. The earlier hinged prostheses (Walldius, Shiers) have been largely superseded by a wide range of devices, many of which are merely surface replacements without intra-medullary bone stems, since these devices mimic the normal action of the joint and are not associated with the earlier problems of difficult wound closure, infection and loosening. The large number of such devices (Attenborough, Deane, Freeman-Swanson, Geomedic, Sheehan) and their relatively short follow-up means that none has yet proved to be superior to the others (Plate 12/6). However, the early results are encouraging with 80 to 90 per cent of patients achieving good results with a low incidence of complications.

In the postoperative management after synovectomy and arthro-plasty there is always a conflict between the need for immobility in a firm compression bandage to achieve haemostatis, wound closure and joint stability and the need for early mobilisation to achieve a rapid return of knee movement and early discharge and to avoid the necessity for later manipulation under anaesthesia (Fig. 12/1). Many surgeons advocate keeping the knee in full extension for four to five days, when modest flexion is then encouraged and full mobilisation with weight-bearing only after stitch removal and the regaining of adequate quadriceps control, usually at 12 to 14 days.

We have found the following programme to be superior. Wound closure is done in 90° of flexion and pressure bandages are applied in this position with the knee supported on three or four pillows. Twenty-four hours postoperatively, strong analgesics are given, all the bandages are removed and the leg is straightened as far as possible, usually to within 15° of full extension. The leg remains straight for 10 to 15 minutes while static quadriceps contractions are encouraged. The leg is then flexed back to 80° and the bandages reapplied. This is repeated on the next three days for gradually increasing lengths of time. By the third day, the leg should be straight and a good quadriceps contraction obtained. On the fifth day, the pressure bandage is removed and the leg straightened. Thereafter, it is only necessary to flex the knee two or three times a day to maintain a good range of motion, so the knee is kept straight and attention focussed on building up quadriceps strength. Weight-bearing can commence as soon as there is control of the knee. The incidence of delayed wound healing is no greater than when more usual methods are employed. Using this method there is no need to manipulate the knee joint under

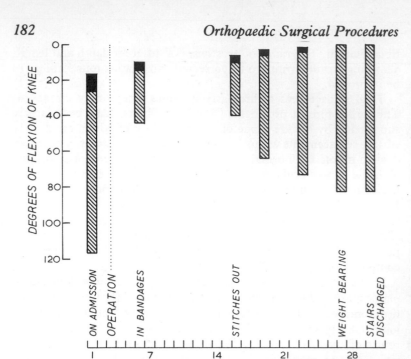

Fig. 12/1 A simple method of recording the flexion deformity, the extension lag (represented by the black parts of the bars) and the range of flexion in the knee joint. Similar charts can be used for any joints

anaesthesia to gain sufficient flexion and the period in hospital is reduced to an average of three weeks, both decided advantages.

If, with other treatment regimes, a manipulation under anaesthesia is deemed necessary, it must not be performed too late or the benefit will be minimal. So, if there is significantly less than 60 to 70° of flexion after three to four weeks, a manipulation is indicated. Pain can be best controlled and a better final result achieved if the joint is supported in the fully flexed position during the first 24 hours and a series of ice packs applied. Movement through to full extension is allowed on the second post-manipulation day.

OSTEOTOMY

High tibial osteotomy if accurately carried out will relieve pain in three-quarters of patients with osteoarthrosis, particularly those with a varus deformity. Patients with rheumatoid arthritis usually have some involvement of both medial and lateral joint compartments and since they more commonly have a valgus than a varus angular deformity the results are rather disappointing. Benjamin (1969), has described a double osteotomy with division of both tibia and femur. The operation might be expected to produce changes in venous blood flow in bone but is probably less useful in correcting angular deformities. In consequence the results, particularly in the hands of those inexperienced in the technique, are disappointing. Any osteotomy of the knee requires up to six weeks in plaster of Paris, although it is usually possible to mobilise the patient within a few days of the operation. Following removal of the cylinder movement is regained quickly and manipulation under anaesthesia is seldom required. However, many patients take up to six months to gain full function.

ARTHRODESIS

Arthrodesis of the knee joint is usually performed by the Charnley compression technique and is a very reliable operation. However, up to three months immobilisation in plaster of Paris is required, one of them non-weight-bearing. Arthrodesis should be used with caution particularly in younger patients and those with rheumatoid arthritis in whom the operation may accentuate the rate of damage in the other major lower limb joints and eventually become a functional handicap. Prevention of damage to the contra-lateral knee depends upon the development and maintenance of strong quadriceps muscles around this knee and a correct raise to the shoe on the side of the arthrodesis. The great advantage of the operation is a production of a pain-free, stable limb. Thus many surgeons tend to combine arthroplasty of one knee joint with arthrodesis of the contra-lateral more severely damaged joint. Such an approach has merit, provided that the patient has been shown capable of coping with a stiff, straight limb in the home by the use of some form of knee splint or brace.

PATELLECTOMY

Patellectomy tends to cause quadriceps weakness and should only be performed in patients with severe osteoarthrosis of the patello-femoral joint; it is rarely required in patients with rheumatoid arthritis. Post-operative management concentrates upon regaining full quadriceps function since joint flexion is rarely compromised. The operation is occasionally performed on patients with severe and persistent chondromalacia.

MENISCECTOMY

Meniscectomy is less commonly employed than previously since a more accurate assessment of the extent of the damage is possible without arthrotomy, using arthrography and arthroscopy. Further, follow-up studies have clearly shown that meniscectomy leads to early osteoarthrosis and should be avoided if possible. The postoperative regimes for knee arthroplasty can be used after meniscectomy, although earlier weight-bearing is often possible.

Hip

Operative treatment of hip disease in almost any type of arthritis should be by total hip replacement. There is little justification, except in the face of sepsis or loosening of a prosthesis, for undertaking earlier operations such as synovectomy, osteotomy, excision or cup arthroplasty. Arthrodesis can be used in osteoarthrosis, particularly in younger patients. It guarantees total and permanent freedom from pain at the expense of mobility but must only be used in cases of unilateral disease where the surrounding joints, knee and lumbar spine, are not involved. Excision arthroplasty of the hip (Girdlestone pseud-arthrosis) is rarely used as a primary procedure, but is valuable as a salvage procedure when there is sepsis or when other operations have failed. The resulting joint is rather unstable and there may be leg shortening of up to 2½in (6cm). It is useful when quick pain relief and increased range of movement is required for patients confined to a wheelchair.

Total hip replacement offers patients a 90 per cent chance of painless movement, but the final range of movement may be less in rheumatoid patients due to permanent soft tissue changes. Prostheses with a metal femoral component and a plastic acetabular component, such as that designed by Charnley and modified by others, are preferred, as these produce less friction than metal on metal devices and there is therefore less chance of later complications (Plate 12/7). Some surgeons remove the greater trochanter to facilitate the operation and then refix it with wire or screws to correct the common adduction deformity. The approach to the hip joint in surgery may be antero-lateral, lateral or posterior, but the general principles of postoperative treatment are similar for each. Non-weight-bearing movements are encouraged from the first or second day, particular attention being paid to the abductors, so as to prevent or minimise any limp once weight-bearing commences. A balance sling or an abduction pillow with the patient free in bed are used to keep the patient in a position where dislocation is less likely. Flexion-rotation movements are the most likely to cause dislocation, so the patient must be warned of this possibility and told to avoid sitting on low toilets, chairs and beds, etc., and crossing the legs, especially during the first few weeks. Flexion is encouraged with a slippery board. Immediate weight-

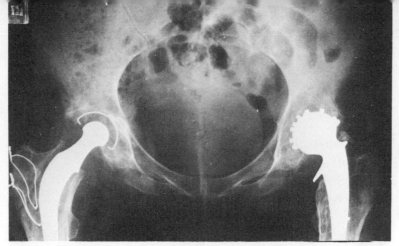

Plate 12/7 Radiograph showing bilateral total hip replacement. The McKee-Farrar prosthesis has metal components, while the more widely used Charnley prosthesis has a polyethylene acetabular component. The marker wire shows the alignment of the component and allows the rate of wear to be calculated. The 'Mexican hat' is placed in the base of a drill hole used for cement fixation. As part of the operation the greater trochanter has been removed and wired back in place

bearing is possible, but is usually delayed until at least the second day, though five to seven days is the usual time. Gait re-education is of paramount importance as the patient will often have walked very poorly prior to the operation, but this will be difficult without reasonable muscle strength and range of movement. Thus specific exercises and daily living activities such as walking, dressing and climbing stairs, must be taught concurrently.

Shoulder

Any operative procedure on the shoulder joint is liable to induce capsulitis (frozen shoulder) with persisting postoperative pain and considerable difficulty in encouraging the return of movement. In consequence there is as yet no satisfactory procedure for the shoulder joint. Excision of the acromion and the underlying bursa relieves pain and improves movement, but often at the expense of joint stability. Arthrodesis of the shoulder may improve upper limb function if the optimum position for fusion is chosen after careful examination and assessment, usually 45° of abduction and 30° of flexion. Prolonged immobilisation of both the shoulder and the elbow is necessary, possibly up to three months, so in rheumatoid patients this operation may be contra-indicated. Good function of the other shoulder and both elbows is also required for a successful arthrodesis. Replacement of the humeral head (Neers prosthesis) is rarely used and probably

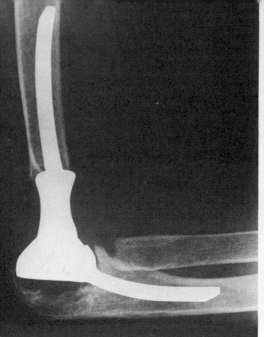

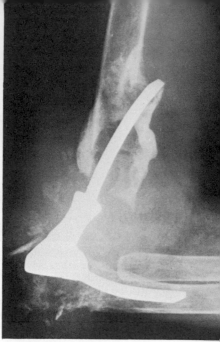

Plate 12/8 Postoperative radiograph of a Dee total elbow replacement

Plate 12/9 Radiograph of the same patient in Plate 12/8 taken four years later showing migration of the humeral component and gross destruction of the joint

relieves pain rather than increasing movement. There are an increasing number of total shoulder prostheses of widely differing design available. However, the operations are technically difficult and may only relieve pain having no effect upon an already limited range of movement. The results of longer term follow-up, particularly the incidence of complications including loosening, are keenly awaited.

Elbow

Synovectomy in a rheumatoid patient can be useful, particularly when combined with excision of the radial head. The range of pain-free movement can be increased, especially of hinge motion, at the expense of joint stability but this is rarely important as these patients have reduced requirements. In osteoarthrosis removal of loose bodies from the joint often dramatically improves movement by removing the mechanical block. In a few patients with both rheumatoid arthritis and osteoarthrosis there is severe damage of the humeral-ulnar compartment and as yet the surgical treatment is unsatisfactory. In some incidences the insertion of a strip of fascia lata will achieve a reasonable range of pain-free movement. There are various types of metal or plastic hinge arthroplasties available, all involving quite drastic excision of the ends of the humerus and ulna. Early results suggested that a stable, pain-free joint with increased movement would result but experience has shown that, due to the constrained nature of the replacement joint, loosening of the stems will occur with ensuing joint instability and increased pain (Plates 12/8 and 12/9). Salvaging a failed elbow arthroplasty is extremely difficult and there is often a gap of up to 3in between the bone ends making fusion impossible, and so some form of external splint is required. New designs for elbow joints that require less bone removal and are less constrained, so imposing less stress on the bones, are being evaluated.

Wrist and Tendon Sheaths

In rheumatoid arthritis surgery is frequently combined with synovectomy of the tendon sheaths. Synovectomy of the wrist and flexor tendons may also be combined with decompression of the median nerve in the carpal tunnel. Median nerve compression symptoms are very common in the early phases of rheumatoid arthritis and may require surgical treatment. Median nerve decompression may be required when other causes are responsible including osteoarthrosis.

Synovectomy of the dorsum of the wrist should always include synovectomy of the related extensor tendons and usually excision of the lower end of ulna (Plates 12/10 and 12/11). The main indications for this operation, which is among the most successful undertaken for rheumatoid arthritis, includes reduced hand and wrist function due to persistent pain in the distal radio-ulnar joint and evidence of extensor

Plate 12/10 Pre-operative radiograph of a rheumatoid wrist showing widening and erosions of the distal radio-ulnar joint due to synovitis

Plate 12/11 Radiograph of the same wrist as Plate 12/10, after excision of the lower end of the ulna

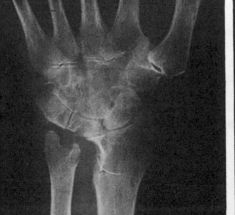
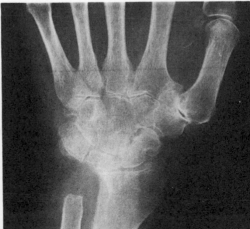

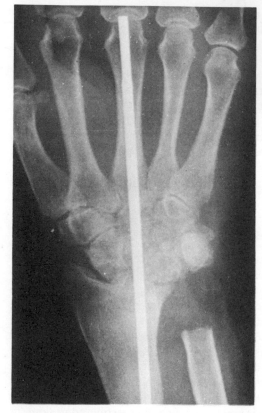

Plate 12/12 Radiograph showing wrist fusion by internal fixation, in rheumatoid arthritis

tendon rupture, stretching or weakness. The operation results in relief of pain and a modest increase in movement of the distal radio-ulnar joint with consequent improvement in hand function in over 90 per cent of patients. There is no evidence of any loss of stability at the wrist and indeed both the head of the radius and the lower end of ulna can be excised in the same forearm without loss of stability, perhaps due to the limited demand of most rheumatoid arthritics.

Arthrodesis of the more severely damaged wrist produces very satisfactory results particularly when patients have only a limited range of painful wrist movements. A variety of techniques for wrist arthrodesis exist, either using plaster of Paris alone to hold the wrist position or combined with internal fixation (Plate 12/12). Most patients find that arthrodesis in a neutral position or in a few degrees of flexion is most satisfactory, particularly for toilet purposes, rather than the usually recommended 10° of extension. Replacement arthroplasty at the wrist is as yet in an early phase of development and it is doubtful whether it will ever have wide usage when the simpler existing techniques produce such satisfactory results.

TENDON REPAIRS

Flexor tendons rarely rupture although the sheaths may require clearance because of diffuse pain and impaired movement at the wrist, in the palm where nodules are particularly apt to develop and in the fingers. Active movement is encouraged from the first postoperative day. Rupture of the extensor tendons is more common although adequate prophylactic surgery should usually prevent rupture. With rupture of the extensor tendons to the index and little fingers, the simplest and most satisfactory results are produced by joining the ruptured tendon to the others. Rupture of the extensor pollicis longus tendon is treated by transfer of extensor indicis proprius. Tendon repair is followed by plaster of Paris support for some three weeks postoperatively when finger movement can be encouraged with the use of a dorsal dynamic splint.

Fingers

In the fingers of rheumatoid patients, peri-articular, tendon and muscle involvement as well as joint disease, contribute to the symptoms and to the characteristic ulnar deviation, swan neck and boutonnière deformities. In addition to synovectomy of the metacarpal and proximal interphalangeal joints, soft tissue release, repair of the extensor apparatus and realignment of the tendons may be required. Although such procedures produce cosmetically satisfactory results, there is usually some loss of movement and finger function is not always improved.

Many surgeons prefer to delay operating until more extensive changes have taken place, often with subluxation of the metacarpophalangeal joints, since an improvement in function is then achieved. A wide range of other soft tissue procedures can be undertaken to correct other hand deformities.

However, in all hand surgery it is most important to undertake a practical assessment of hand function to determine the patient's real wishes and needs. Subsequent surgery must be planned on a very individual basis to ensure that the patient's demands will be met as there is a real risk that in improving or restoring one function, another of equal importance is lost. Thus, in simple terms, it is often very difficult to combine both a good grip and good pinch movement and some surgeons will elect to provide one function in each hand.

There are various types of prosthesis available particularly for the metacarpophalangeal joints (Swanson, Calnan-Nichol, etc) but none of them are entirely satisfactory (Plates 12/13 and 12/14). They straighten the fingers but only allow approximately 25° of movement, so if the patient has this range of movement available pre-operatively, she is unlikely to be happy with the result, unless pain relief and improved appearance are the aims. Good movement of the other joints of the fingers is a necessity if a good functional result is to be achieved. Many of these finger joint replacements have a tendency to slip or disintegrate; if this happens, salvage can leave the patient in a worse position functionally than before surgery was started. The post-operative management varies considerably, some surgeons keeping the joint in extension with plaster support for 10 to 14 days, while others encourage early flexion. Once movement is allowed, a lively splint which keeps the resting joints in extension and encourages active flexion against resistance is useful (Plate 12/15).

Arthrodesis of a painful, deformed or unstable proximal interphalangeal joint of the fingers and interphalangeal and metacarpophalangeal joints of the thumb in the rheumatoid and of the carpo-metacarpal joint of the thumb in the osteoarthrotic patient, will correct deformity and may substantially improve pinch movements and relieve pain. Arthrodesis is achieved by K-wires and immobilisation in plaster or by the insertion of a small polypropylene peg without plaster support. Degenerative changes in the carpo-metacarpal joint of the thumb can also be treated by excision of the trapezium. The gap

Plate 12/13 Radiograph of a hand with severe rheumatoid arthritis showing destruction and subluxation of the metacarpophalangeal joints with ulnar deviation

Plate 12/14 Radiograph of the same hand in Plate 12/13 after replacement of the metacarpophalangeal joints with Swanson silastic prostheses

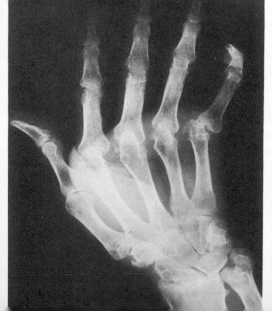
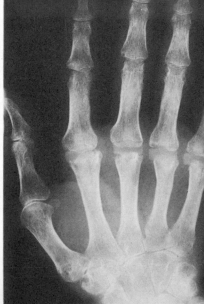

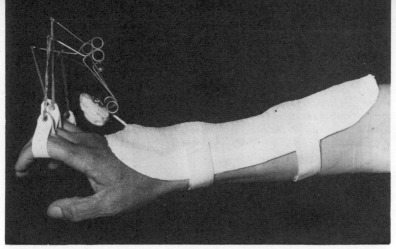

Plate 12/15 A lively splint allows finger flexion against the resistance of springs and the supporting elastic bands

left can either be allowed to fill with fibrous tissue or be filled with a silastic prosthesis or silicone rubber sponge.

REFERENCE

Benjamin, A. (1969). 'Double osteotomy for the painful knee in rheumatoid arthritis and osteoarthritis.' *Journal of Bone and Joint Surgery*, **51B**, 694.

BIBLIOGRAPHY

Boyle, J. A., and Buchanan, W. W. (1971). *Clinical Rheumatology*. Blackwell Scientific Publications.

Copeman's Textbook of Rheumatic Diseases. Ed. J. T. Scott (1977). Churchill Livingstone.

Goble, R. E. A. and Nichols, P. J. R. (1971). *Rehabilitation of the Severely Disabled, Vol. 1, Evaluation of a Disabled Living Unit; Vol. 2, Management*. Butterworths.

Hollander, J. L., and McCarty, D. J. (Jt. eds. 1972). *Arthritis and Allied Conditions: A Textbook of Rheumatology*. Lea & Febiger, Philadelphia.

Hughes, G. R. V. (1976). *Modern Topics in Rheumatology*. William Heinemann Medical Books Ltd.

Hughes, G. R. V. (1977). *Connective Tissue Diseases*. Blackwell Scientific Publications.

Mason, M. and Currey, H. L. F. (Jt. eds. 1976). *An Introduction to Clinical Rheumatology*. Pitman Medical.

Medicine, Third series, 'Issues 12, 13 and 14, December 1978–February 1979. Medical Education (International) Ltd., Oxford.

Equipment for the Disabled; a supplement on Wheelchairs and Outdoor Transport. Published and obtainable from The National Fund for Research into Crippling Diseases, 2, Foredown Drive, Portslade, Brighton BN4 2BB.

See also the Bibliography at the end of Chapters 13 and 14.

ACKNOWLEDGEMENT

Dr. A. G. Mowat, Mrs. J. M. Abery and Mr. C. P. Roberts wish to thank their colleagues in the medical team at Oxford for advice and encouragement. They are particularly grateful to Mrs. Sheila Strudwick for typing the chapters; to Mr. R. Emanuel for the photographs and to Mr. G. R. Bartlett, DIP.C.D. for Fig. 8/1.

Chapter 13

Non-Articular Pain

by C. M. MARSHALL, M.C.S.P., DIP.T.P.

The most common reason people seek medical aid is for the relief of
certain symptoms, but it should be borne in mind that there are
sometimes other reasons as well – such as the need for help with a
disability, reassurance, sympathy or the desire for compensation
following some specific incident. The source of their symptoms may
be articular or non-articular. For the purposes of this chapter, structures which are not of bone or cartilage will be assumed to be
non-articular. Therefore, pure articular conditions such as arthritis,
arthroses and fractures will not be considered, but rather some of the
more common non-articular lesions which are the cause of the
patient's chief symptom, pain.

EXAMINATION OF THE PATIENT

It is the duty of all physiotherapists to examine their patients
thoroughly so that a clear picture is obtained of the symptoms, which
is then matched with comparable signs. There can be no substitute for
this routine accurate examination, for without it there is no means of
applying treatment to the faulty structures, except on a 'hit or miss'
basis, or of assessing progress, be it improvement or deterioration. A
basic routine, with subjective examination preceding objective, is
suggested (see p. 205).

When the patient is first referred for treatment it is often easiest to
seek a clear picture of his present symptoms prior to the overall history
of the condition. The precise area and behaviour of pain being known,
the irritability of the condition can be estimated, so that during the
objective examination there is neither over- nor under-examination of
relevant structures and exacerbation of pain is thus minimised, but
comparable signs are not overlooked. The character of the pain
described by the patient can also be helpful. True muscle pain is

exacerbated by exercise, is usually diffuse and is often referred, with distribution following a spinal segmental pattern and associated with referred tenderness of the deep structures, while periosteum, fascia, tendon sheaths and skin give accurately localised pain which is often burning in character. Functional limitations of the patient should be ascertained and the dominance of pain or stiffness imposing them noted.

The objective examination should be subdivided into active and passive movements. Initially general posture is observed and obvious muscle wasting looked for. Then all muscles and joints underlying, or able to refer pain to the area of pain complained of, and therefore previously ascertained by questioning the patient, must be examined. Movements that reproduce or alter the symptoms are noted. If movements are found to be limited the range obtainable should be measured and recorded and any abnormality of scapulohumeral movement noted. If movements appear to be full and painless then a moderate degree of pressure is applied at the limit of range in order to confirm that this is so. During active movement both contractile structures (muscle) and inert structures (joint capsule, ligaments, bursae) move, whereas true passive movement is produced by an outside force so that no muscle contraction occurs. Pain from contractile structures occurs on contraction so that it may be necessary to confirm a muscle lesion by strongly resisted isometric contractions – thus eliminating inert structures. Pain from inert structures occurs on stretching or pressure and it must be decided from the pattern of painful passive movement obtained whether all the inert structures limiting movement at a joint are involved (i.e. a diffuse capsular lesion) or only a small part of them (e.g. a ligament). The examination should not be limited to passive physiological movements but should also include the accessory movements obtainable in the joints under consideration (Maitland, 1977). Any muscle weakness should be noted and recorded using the Oxford scale, as should any alteration of normal tone. For more widespread muscle involvement the use of a standard muscle chart is recommended for recording the information. Palpation will reveal any localised warmth which will indicate an active lesion, and any areas of localised tenderness, thickening or swelling.

THE SHOULDER AREA

There are many causes of pain in the shoulder. The pain may arise due to intrinsic disease of the glenohumeral joint, pathology in the periarticular structures or from disease in the spine, chest or abdominal viscera. Initial examination including mapping out the area of pain, as already suggested, will give a useful guide as to where the source lies. When the patient is complaining of predominantly shoulder pain rather than neck-shoulder radiating pains, it is usually indicative of pathology in the glenohumeral joint or its peri-articular structures. However, most shoulder lesions produce some referred pain into the area of the insertion of the deltoid muscle.

Although the shoulder should be regarded clinically as an area rather than a single joint, due to the number of patients whose pain does arise from some distant structure, only the most common local non-articular causes will be considered here.

Apart from acute traumatic lesions, 90 per cent of painful disabilities of the shoulder are due to acute or chronic tendinitis and bursitis, lesions of the musculo-tendinous cuff and adhesive capsulitis. Arthritis of the shoulder joint causes less than 5 per cent of painful shoulders, apart from patients suffering from generalised arthropathies (Zanca, 1971). The reason for this is due to the anatomical arrangement, in that the glenohumeral joint depends for stability largely on the tendons that surround it rather than the shallow glenoid cavity and remarkably loose joint capsule. The long head of biceps tends to hold the humeral head into the glenoid cavity while the capsule is strengthened by the flattened expansions superiorly of supraspinatus, anteriorly of subscapularis and posteriorly by infraspinatus and teres minor, or in other words, the rotator cuff. It is also strengthened below by the long head of triceps – although not so closely as in other parts of the rotator cuff, as here capsule and muscle are separated by the axillary nerve and posterior circumflex humeral vessels. Therefore, this inferior part of the capsule, which on abduction of the arm is tightly stretched over the head of the humerus, may be subjected to the greatest strain.

Degenerative Tendinitis

Progressive degenerative changes in the structure of the rotator cuff have been noted, even in people with no symptoms, particularly after middle age. The supraspinatus tendon is most frequently affected, probably due to the position of its insertion on the highest part of the tuberosity of the humerus. This renders it particularly subject to minor trauma as it impinges on the acromion and coraco-acromial ligament during abduction with the arm medially rotated. Due to this mechanical stress and strain, and consequent low-grade inflammation, degeneration becomes more marked, the tendon shows signs of thinning and weakness and it becomes stretched – thus being more likely to be caught as the humerus swings under the coraco-acromial arch. The subacromial (subdeltoid) bursa, because of its situation, is also frequently involved in this type of lesion and may shrink with varying degrees of fibrosis. Bony changes may develop later due to the gradual degenerative process. These may take the form of sclerosis, eburnation or minute cyst formation seen in the head of the humerus (Bateman, 1972).

The patient complains initially of a catching type of discomfort in the shoulder, of insidious onset with no precipitating incident, particularly on lifting the arm. Limitation of movement gradually occurs. The pain grows into a persistent gnawing ache radiating down the outside of the arm and forearm, which causes difficulty in sleeping and from which he can gain no relief. On examination about 70° active abduction is possible without pain. There is usually a painful arc of movement between 70 and 120° abduction (similarly in adduction) which is more pronounced on active than passive movement. Obviously some structure must be pinched in this position, the supraspinatus tendon being the most common but also the subacromial bursa, and tendons of infraspinatus or subscapularis being other possibilities. In order to differentiate, it will be found that resisted abduction is painful if supraspinatus is the cause, resisted lateral rotation if infraspinatus and resisted medial rotation if subscapularis. Should the bursa be the inflamed area, then the painful arc is often the only sign found, isometric contractions proving painless. The longer the lesion has been neglected, the more likely the shoulder to have become frozen, probably due to general disinclination to use the painful arm, and thus limitation of movements may be found.

AIMS OF TREATMENT

These should be the relief of pain and preservation of joint movement so that 'freezing' is avoided. In order to relieve pain the affected tendon or bursa may be injected with local anaesthetic and/or corticosteroids, and appropriate drugs may be prescribed (Chapter 15). The physiotherapist may apply ice to the whole of the painful shoulder and shoulder girdle area by means of an ice pack, or frequently changed damp towels with ice fragments clinging to them, in order both to relieve pain and to obtain muscle relaxation. It should be remembered that in order to be effective the ice must cover the affected muscles from origin to insertion. This should be done prior to careful exercise designed to maintain and improve range, but avoiding movements that are known to cause pain. Pendular movements with a weight of approximately 1kg tied to the wrist and the patient comfortably positioned so that the trunk is horizontal (i.e. either prone lying or forward leaning) are often found helpful at first, especially if the patient is given time to relax in this position prior to any attempt at movement. Pure glenohumeral movement with a minimum of effort is thus obtained. Progression is by way of free active movements and then, if possible, resisted work in order to build up general strength in unaffected muscles, but all the time avoiding as far as possible that part of the range which causes pain. Localised ultra-sound, pulsed in order to avoid any heating effect, to the site of the lesion is sometimes found to be of value.

If the condition is at the early stage of localised tendinitis with no limitation of movement, massage in the form of deep transverse frictions to the offending portion of tendon should be accurately applied and the previously described treatments will be unnecessary. Treatment for frozen shoulder is described separately (see p. 200).

Calcific Tendinitis

Calcified deposits may occur in the tendon substance of supraspinatus and less frequently in that of infraspinatus, subscapularis and teres minor. The reason for the change in tendon substance is still not established although it is possible that abnormal ageing of collagen fibres may initiate the calcification mechanism. Deposits may be present for years, remaining within the tendon, under no tension and without causing trouble, so that if discovered by chance on the radiograph for some unrelated condition, they should be ignored. However, symptoms are caused if the tendon is irritated so that the deposit enlarges under pressure within the tendon and so impinges under the coraco-acromial arch during abduction. This may occur as an acute episode of rapid onset, with constant acute pain inhibiting sleep and accentuated by any arm movement, actual or anticipated, or isometric muscle contraction, so that there is gross apparent limitation of movement due to pain and muscle spasm. During this stage the shoulder may be warm and swollen. When subacute, the pain is referred to the area of deltoid insertion and the limitation will be found to be an arc of about 70 to 100° abduction. There is little relation between the size of the deposit and the severity of symptoms. Inflammatory changes may also develop in the subacromial bursa. Occasionally spontaneous rupture of the deposit into the bursa may occur, relieving the tension in the tendon and so the symptoms.

TREATMENT

In the acute stage this is initially conservative, aiming to relieve pain by the use of analgesic-anti-inflammatory drugs and resting the arm in a sling usually worn under the clothes. During this stage, a treatment regime of ice pack, then ultra-sound (pulsed) around the area of calcification as shown on the radiograph, followed by a further ice pack over the area may be used. The ultra-sound should be localised to the precise area of calcification as soon as the pain subsides sufficiently to permit this. Movement should be encouraged at the earliest opportunity but any movement that places the tendon on a stretch, e.g. extension or extension and lateral rotation if supraspinatus is affected, should be avoided. With improvement (i.e. less pain) exercises may be progressed by frequency and change of starting position and finally by the use of resistance. If improvement does not occur rapidly, the continuing acute pain predisposes to frozen shoulder, so that occasionally surgical removal of the deposit, which provides dramatic relief, becomes the treatment of choice. Following this, movement should be begun as soon as pain allows and exercises continued until normal range and power is achieved in the shoulder.

Ruptures of the Rotator Cuff

It has already been stated that progressive degenerative changes are known to occur in the rotator cuff structures. These may lead to gradual thinning of the cuff, which eventually wears through, or some minor incident such as a fall on the outstretched hand may precipitate it. Alternatively rupture may occur following dislocation of the shoulder. The patient experiences an initial sharp pain in the shoulder and the arm feels limp and useless. This is followed by dull aching of the joint area which steadily increases so that interference with sleep occurs. Pain is usually the predominant complaint and it may be referred down the arm and to the neck. Joint stiffness develops gradually due to continued inability to lift the arm. If the rupture is only partial, then the signs are less definite; pain is less but there is some loss of power and range of abduction. Arthrography may be used to determine the exact site and extent of the tear.

TREATMENT

Surgical repair may be considered if the tear is very large but the majority of patients obtain satisfactory use of the arm with good conservative treatment. The pain is mainly due to the inflammatory reaction in the torn cuff and subacromial bursa, and for this reason the arm should be rested at the beginning of treatment. However, finger, wrist and elbow exercises together with isometric work for deltoid and non-painful muscles of the cuff, should be commenced immediately, followed by pendular movements as soon as possible. As the pain subsides assisted active movements are introduced and gradually progressed to resisted exercises using normal patterns of movement. It is important to strengthen the accessory muscles of the shoulder, such as biceps and triceps, in order to replace the now inefficient cuff. It is thought that in some patients good range of movement in the shoulder is due to adhesions between the deltoid muscle and thickened subacromial bursa which is also adherent to the rotator cuff especially about the site of rupture (Meviaser, 1971).

The Biceps Tendon

The long head of biceps arises by a long tendon from the supraglenoid tubercle within the capsule of the shoulder joint. It arches over the head of the humerus and emerges from the joint by passing behind the transverse humeral ligament. It is this ligament that is responsible for retaining it in the bicipital groove, and should it rupture, usually due to injury, the tendon will slip in and out of the groove during movement and a painful snapping sensation will be felt. There will also be an associated capsular tear. Inflammatory changes and therefore pain are thus initiated and the patient becomes unwilling to use the arm, the capsule contracts and limitation of movement occurs. On palpation the tendon is usually tender, particularly over the bicipital groove. It should, however, be remembered that most patients will find that firm pressure over the tendon is uncomfortable, and experience is needed in the correct technique. Conservative treatment should consist of avoiding movements where the tendon is under strong tension, particularly in abduction and external rotation. Pure glenohumeral movement may be retained by pendular movements of the weighted arm as previously described, first taking care to obtain good relaxation of the arm and shoulder girdle by allowing it to hang in the dependent position for at least 10 minutes. As pain subsides, so muscle power of the arm may be built up with progressive resistance exercises, but still avoiding those movements that put the tendon under strong tension.

Degenerative changes may occur during middle age similar to those of the rotator cuff. The tendon frays and the synovial sheath becomes inflamed. On examination there is often pain on resisted flexion of the elbow with supination and tenderness to palpation over the tendon. Symptoms may be precipitated by jerky lifting with outstretched arms or unaccustomed exercises such as the first game of tennis of the season.

Treatment should aim at reducing the inflammation of the sheath, preventing adhesion formation and maintaining full range of shoulder

movements. Thus the tendon may be injected with local anaesthetic
and/or corticosteroids (see Chapter 15) and then gentle active exercises should be instituted. Alternatively localised transverse frictions
are often beneficial.

Complete rupture of the biceps tendon may occur following
trauma. A bulge is noticed in the front of the arm and pressure over
the bicipital groove is painful. Elbow flexion is only slightly weak, but
the biceps is noted to be ineffective. In most cases, general strengthening of the arm will give good functional use. However, if the patient is
young and needs the arm specifically to earn his living, then surgery
may be necessary.

Frozen Shoulder (Adhesive Capsulitis)

This is a term that is widely used to describe a syndrome resulting
from many diverse pathologies. Although there is a small group where
the cause is idiopathic, a frozen shoulder generally results as a reaction
to immobility of the arm due to pain, fear or abnormal muscle tone. It
is noticed that disuse of the arm in a tense, over-anxious patient with a
low pain threshold pre-disposes to this syndrome, and that older
patients are more susceptible. It can thus be appreciated that any of
the previously described conditions could initiate a frozen shoulder,
as well as referred pain from cardiac, gall bladder, diaphragm or
cervical spine lesions.

It has been suggested by many investigators that psychological
factors may pre-dispose to the development of a frozen shoulder, but a
recent study does not support this view (Wright and Haq, 1975).
However the finding of a much increased incidence of the tissue
antigen HLA–B27 offers some support to the concept of genetic
influences in up to half the patients (Bulgen, Hazleman and Voak,
1976). Others have noted an increased incidence in diabetics.

The patient will complain of pain in the shoulder region which may
radiate up to the neck and down the arm. The shoulder is stiff, usually
progressively so, and glenohumeral movement is limited in all ranges
although this may vary according to the aetiology. The normally loose
glenohumeral joint capsule becomes thickened and contracted, losing
its folds inferiorly as they become glued together. The synovial membrane becomes stuck to the articular cartilage, the subacromial bursa
may shrink and surrounding muscles show protective spasm due to
pain, and therefore waste.

TREATMENT

There is no doubt that the most important part of treatment is preventive by discovering and effectively treating the primary cause as early as possible, and explaining to the patient the importance of maintaining the range of movement. In the small group of patients where the cause is idiopathic, fortunately, the condition usually recovers spontaneously although this may take up to two years.

However, a large number of patients with frozen shoulders of varying degrees from varying causes are referred for physiotherapy. The aim of treatment must be to relieve pain and improve the range of movement so that they have as good and functional an arm as possible. One effective method of treatment is that suggested by Maitland (1977), using the appropriate grade and combination of accessory and physiological passive movements according to whether pain or stiffness dominate. Alternatively, there are many advocates for a regime using ice and relaxation techniques, which may be by means of suspension or pendular exercises, or those of proprioceptive neuromuscular facilitation techniques. Once pain is subsiding and range of movement improving then appropriate muscle strengthening techniques may be incorporated in the treatment, remembering that they should only be used in the pain-free range available. Sometimes manipulation under anaesthetic is undertaken in the later stages and when this procedure is used it is important that the physiotherapist should be in the theatre to observe the range of movement achieved, for it will be her job to encourage and assist the patient to maintain it afterwards, despite initial soreness.

Although individual therapists will undoubtedly achieve good results with one or other method, it must be appreciated that comparative studies do not show that any method of treatment is superior and that physiotherapy, if badly applied, may make the pain worse (Hazleman, 1972). Finally, although the patient should be reassured that full function will return, careful measurement shows that there is a small, permanent loss of range of movement (Clarke, Willis, Fish and Nichols, 1975).

For use of analgesics and/or local injections of anaesthetic and corticosteroid, see Chapter 15.

THE ELBOW AREA

Tennis Elbow

This is probably one of the most common causes of pain at the lateral side of the elbow. It is important that the pain is differentiated from that due to cervical spondylosis; this may be difficult as the conditions not infrequently co-exist. The condition is usually found in people over 30 years of age and it is caused by repetitive movements at the elbow region, especially pronation and supination or forced extension, not necessarily by playing tennis.

The onset of pain is usually gradual, accentuated by the use of the arm and improved with rest. Radiation of pain to the muscles of the forearm may occur and, if severe, will inhibit gripping. On examination there is pain over the lateral epicondylar area of the humerus on active wrist extension, particularly with radial deviation and with the elbow in extension. Passive elbow extension, especially in adduction, is limited in the last few degrees if examined carefully, with an end feel of elastic resistance. An area of tenderness can usually be accurately located, the most common site being over the lateral ligament or slightly anterior to it.

There have been many different views expressed as to the pathology of this lesion. Mostly it is thought to be due to minor strain in the region of the common extensor origin and, many authorities now say, of extensor carpi radialis brevis in particular. It has been suggested that a small number of resistant cases could be due to an entrapment neuropathy of the radial nerve as it passes over the fibrous edge of extensor carpi radialis brevis and then goes deep into the supinator muscle. When the extensor origin tightens it can compress the radial nerve and thus the symptoms are reproduced by extension and radial deviation of the wrist with elbow extension. In others there may be chondromalacia of the radial head cartilage.

TREATMENT

Initially treatment is usually by injection of corticosteroid mixed with local anaesthetic, into the site of maximum tenderness (see Chapter 15). Repeated injections may be required. Patients referred for physiotherapy are most effectively treated by deep transverse frictions localised to the most painful part of the tendon, usually for 15 to 20 minutes twice weekly. Ultrasound, again to the appropriate area, has sometimes been found to be of value. All these measures should be accompanied by rest of the extensor muscles of the forearm. Enforced rest in plaster of Paris for two to four weeks is frequently tried but is rarely successful. Heat and other forms of massage give only transitory relief. Should these conservative measures fail, surgical treatment may be required.

Golfer's Elbow

This is a less common but comparable condition to tennis elbow occurring at the medial epicondylar region of the humerus. The lesion occurs at the common flexor tendon origin at the medial epicondyle and on examination the pain can be reproduced by resisted flexion of the wrist with the elbow in extension. Treatment is similar to that for tennis elbow.

PERIPHERAL ENTRAPMENT NEUROPATHIES

Pressure exerted upon a peripheral nerve gives rise to certain well-known symptoms, namely pins and needles which is then followed by pain, numbness and muscle weakness if the pressure is constant and unrelieved. This may be due to mechanical irritation, trauma, or some indeterminate cause which leads to local inflammation and therefore swelling and thus compression.

Carpal Tunnel Syndrome

This common condition is due to compression of the median nerve as it passes with the flexor tendons between the flexor retinaculum and the bones of the carpus. Often there is no apparent cause but it may be associated with trauma, such as a Colles' fracture; or any condition which reduces the size of the carpal tunnel such as arthritis or fluid retention in connective tissue as sometimes occurs, for example, in pregnancy.

The characteristic history is of gradual onset of tingling and pain, followed by numbness of the first three fingers, which may spread up the inner side of the arm. In advanced cases there is slight weakness of the muscles of the thenar eminence particularly abductor pollicis brevis, appropriate median sensory impairment and sometimes some autonomic symptoms in the form of painful swelling of the fingers, discolouration and alteration in sweating. The symptoms are often worse at night, disturbing sleep, and the patient may state that some relief is gained by hanging the arm over the side of the bed. Diagnostically the symptoms can often be reproduced by firmly flexing the wrist for one minute (wrist extension may also be used but the results are not so reliable) or pressure over the flexor retinaculum, thus distinguishing it from referred pain from other causes such as cervical spondylosis and thoracic outlet syndrome. If electrodiagnosis is used there is conduction delay in the median nerve.

TREATMENT

This is aimed at reducing the inflammatory reaction and the physiotherapist may be asked to make a splint to rest the wrist in the neutral position at night – this is often diagnostic in the relief it provides. Injection of a suitable corticosteroid preparation is often successful (see Chapter 15). Should these measures fail the flexor retinaculum is divided surgically and the nerve decompressed.

Morton's Metatarsalgia

This is due to pinching of one of the digital nerves just before it divides to supply the adjacent sides of two toes, most commonly the third and fourth. With continued pressure the nerve becomes oedematous and fibrous thickening, or a neuroma, occurs. There may be a primary acute traumatic cause or it may be due to abnormal hyperextension at the metatarsophalangeal joint due to rheumatoid arthritis, congenital deformity or constant wearing of high-heeled shoes that incline the forefoot down and force hyperextension of the toes. The latter may account for the fact that it is found more commonly in women than men. The patient complains of episodic acute pain in the toes on walking, necessitating removal of the shoe and rubbing the foot. At first there are no symptoms between episodes but with continued pressure dull pain in the metatarsal area may develop. On palpation between the appropriate metatarsal heads, acute pain may be elicited and sensory changes induced in the toes.

TREATMENT

Conservative treatment consists of choosing correctly fitting shoes and wearing a metatarsal pad to prevent hyperextension of the metatarso-phalangeal joint. A metatarsal bar may be attached to the sole of the shoe. Faradic footbaths and exercises do not usually help. If no relief is gained from conservative measures then surgical excision of the neuroma is performed.

Other less frequently encountered entrapment neuropathies occur, such as compression of the tibial nerve beneath the flexor retinaculum below the medial malleolus of the ankle (tarsal tunnel syndrome), of the common peroneal nerve at the neck of the fibula, of the ulnar nerve at the elbow and of the anterior interosseous nerve at the point where it is given off from the median nerve as it passes into the forearm between the two heads of pronator teres (pronator syndrome). Treatment is either conservative by corticosteroid injection or surgical decompression.

'FIBROSITIS'

Many patients complain of pain at sites of tendon insertion, bony prominences or in major muscle masses, and while in most instances careful examination will reveal the source, there are some in whom exhaustive investigation may fail to show any cause. 'Fibrositis' is a vague term describing a condition of pain and stiffness in myofascial structures which is often temporary. The areas involved are usually related to some moving part under stress. There seems little doubt that there are times in a person's life such as bereavement, the menopause, or depression when the threshold of complaint about such pains is lowered. Contributory causes are legion, but common irritants are fatigue, worry, chronic illness and under-nourishment, and these are often augmented by damp, cold or draught. It has been said that these patients keep their muscles as tense as their minds and it may be that this is reaction to chronic strain, poor posture or repeated occupational stress. The most common regions complained of are the neck and shoulders, lumbar and gluteal regions.

On palpation, particularly if the condition is acute, there is usually some muscle spasm as well as general tenderness with certain painful trigger points. These may be nodules which are fibro-fatty or fibrous tissue, and sometimes herniate through the superficial fascia. The reason for the nodules is obscure. The muscles may feel thickened, though exploration has shown little pathological change, but if the condition is of long standing the muscles are more likely to feel stringy and atonic.

TREATMENT

This is aimed at relieving pain, improving the circulation, obtaining muscular relaxation and then strengthening the appropriate muscle groups and good physiotherapy plays an important part. The patient should be fully supported in a comfortable position while some form of superficial heat (such as infra-red irradiation or hot pad) is applied. This should be followed by massage and then isometric postural exercises which may be progressed to resisted exercises later. The actual course of treatment should be short but the patient should be carefully instructed as to the value of home heat (hot bath, shower or lamp) and continuing the exercises. For use of analgesic drugs see Chapter 15.

EXAMINATION FOR NON-ARTICULAR PAIN IN THE SHOULDER REGION

Subjective Examination (by questioning)

1. Map out on body chart precise areas of pain complained of. Indicate types of pain and worst area(s). Show any areas of altered sensation.

2. Note factors exacerbating and relieving pain. For how long?
3. Is sleep interfered with? Can the arm be slept on at night? State of symptoms on rising in morning.
4. Do symptoms impose any functional limitations?
5. Have recent radiographs been taken? Which areas?
6. Is general health good? (So eliminate cardiac, gall bladder or diaphragmatic causes.)
7. What tablets are being taken for this or any other condition?
8. History, i.e. onset and course followed. Now improving, deteriorating or static? Previous history?
9. Any past history of similar symptoms? How treated and result?

Objective Examination (by testing and observation)

1. Posture – head on neck, spine, shoulder levels. Wasting of arm. Localised thickening or swelling.
2. Routine check of all neck movements.
3. Active shoulder movements. Note limitations and any abnormality of scapulohumeral movement, range/pain relationships.
4. Resisted isometric contractions of all muscles underlying areas of pain charted or able to refer pain to these areas.
5. Muscle power of above muscles.
6. Passive physiological shoulder movements – pure movement (e.g. abduction of shoulder joint with scapula fixed). Note range/pain relationship.
7. Passive accessory glenohumeral movements. Check those of the sterno-clavicular and acromio-clavicular joints.
8. Check elbow movements.
9. Check 'case notes' for reports and relevant tests.

Plan Appropriate Treatment

REFERENCES

Bateman, J. E. (1972). *The Shoulder and Neck*. W. B. Saunders.
Bulgen, D. Y., Hazleman, B. L. and Voak. D. (1976). 'HLA–B27 and Frozen Shoulder.' *Lancet*, 1, 1042.
Clarke, G. R., Willis, L. A., Fish, W. W. and Nichols, P. J. R. (1975). 'Preliminary Studies in measuring range of motion in normal and painful stiff shoulders.' *Rheumatology and Rehabilitation*, 14, 39.
Hazleman, B. L. (1972). 'The Painful Stiff Shoulder.' *Rheumatology and Physical Medicine*, 11, 413.
Maitland, G. D. (1977). *Peripheral Manipulation*, 2nd edition. Butterworths.

Meviaser, J. S. (1971). 'Ruptures of the Rotator Cuff of the Shoulder.' *Archives of Surgery*, 102, 483.

Wright, V. and Haq, A. M. M. M. (1976). 'Periarthritis of the shoulder.' *Annals of the Rheumatic Diseases*, 35, 213.

Zanca, P. (1971). 'Shoulder Pain – Involvement of the Acromio-clavicular Joint.' *American Journal of Roentgenology*, 112, 493.

BIBLIOGRAPHY

Cailliet, R. (1966). *Shoulder Pain*. F. A. Davis & Co., Philadelphia.

Johnson, E. W., Hughes, A.C., and Haase, K. H. (1962). 'Carpal Tunnel Syndrome – A Review.' *Archives of Physical Medicine and Rehabilitation*, 43, 420.

Kapell, H. P. and Thompson, W. A. L. (1963). *Peripheral Entrapment Neuropathies*. Williams and Wilkins Co., Baltimore.

Kellgren, J. H. (1938). 'Preliminary Account of Referred Pains Arising from Muscle.' *British Medical Journal*, 1, 325.

Kellgren, J. H. (1938). 'Observations on Referred Pain Arising from Muscle.' *Clinical Science*, 3, 175.

Lewis, T. (1938). 'Suggestions Relating to the Study of Somatic Pain.' *British Medical Journal*, 1, 321.

Melville, L. D. (1972). 'The Differential Diagnosis of Nerve Compression Syndrome in the Hand and Arm.' *The Hand*, 4, (2).

Roles, N. C. and Maudsley, R. H. (1972). 'Radial Tunnel Syndrome.' *Journal of Bone and Joint Surgery*, 54B, (3).

Stewart, I. M. (1972). 'Nerve Entrapment in the Upper Limb.' *The Hand*, 4, (2).

See also the Bibliography at the end of Chapters 12 and 14.

Chapter 14

Principles of Manipulation

by J. HICKLING, M.C.S.P.

An attempt to select principles must be confined to discussion of prime constituents, a search for a general formula. The reader must study the literature of the subject for detailed information about the practice of manipulation, particularly about examination, contraindications, and technique.

The endeavour to crystallise such a formula poses three immediate problems:

1. The definition of the word 'manipulation' is by no means agreed. To take extreme examples: it may be used to describe either the forcing of a painful and limited range of movement under anaesthesia, or a small painless movement on the conscious patient.

2. The purpose of manipulation is also by no means generally agreed; success in treatment being ascribed by different experts to the resolution of different pathologies.

3. A statement of general principles seems to require guidelines about the dangers of manipulation. To do this in the midst of confusion about definition and purpose seemed impossible.

The first concern here, therefore, is with terminology and definitions.

TERMINOLOGY AND DEFINITIONS

All manipulation is passive movement, but not all passive movement can properly be called manipulation. Somewhere along the line, as force, speed, complexity or purpose change, a passive movement becomes a manipulation but there might be disagreement about exactly when this occurs.

The Use of Force

The use of controlled force is essential to manipulation, but the word 'force' is alarming because it has connotations of ruthless intention, lack of control, and provocation of pain.

Terminology in which 'relaxed passive movement' is contrasted with 'forced passive movement' and 'manipulation' carries the suggestion that forced passive movement and manipulation are not relaxed. This in turn suggests that the resistance which is being encountered is that of muscle activity, and an association is often made with the provocation of pain. In fact, of course, the whole art of manipulation lies in having the patient perfectly relaxed, and the resistance that is being overcome is practically never that of muscle activity.

Some re-definition is needed here, and the terms 'free' and 'stressed passive movement' are offered, to be used in the following way:

Force in Normal Movement

Free passive movement is movement in which there is no encounter with tissue resistance at all, and which therefore requires no force for its performance. As soon as there is even the lightest encounter with tissue resistance, the movement is called *stressed passive movement*, necessarily demanding the use of force for its completion.

By the use of the word 'stressed' in this way it is hoped to avoid the rather dire nuances that surround the word 'forced', while emphasising that in most movements in the body, full range can only be achieved by using a degree of force to overcome normal increasing tissue resistance.

The term 'end-feel' is used by Cyriax (1978), to describe the quality of the factor limiting a passive movement, as perceived by the hand. It thus refers to the element of palpation which exists in passive movement, and is related to the term 'tissue tension sense' that is used by manipulators.

There are three 'end-feels' in the normal:

The first is *bone-to-bone*, in which active and passive ranges are equal.

The next two are *tissue approximation* and *tissue tension*, and in both of these, passive range is greater than active. Passive movement into such ranges is partly free and partly stressed, and the point at which the change occurs, i.e. the point of encounter with first tissue resistance, is earlier in the range than is usually recognised.

The term *accessory range* is here used to denote that part of stressed passive movement which lies beyond the end of active movement. The end of active movement lies somewhere beyond the end of free passive movement and before full stressed passive movement.

The relative proportions of free passive movement, active movement, and stressed passive movement vary endlessly in different movements, positions, physiques and ages, as does the resistance offered by the tissues. A general formula may be offered as illustrated in Fig. 14/1.

In the normal, bone-to-bone and tissue approximation are painless. Tissue tension may also be painless, but in some physiques it may be anything from slightly uncomfortable to downright painful in the normal. This must be borne in mind when evaluating the abnormal.

Within the gross primary movements which can be achieved actively there are elements of slide, roll and spin which together

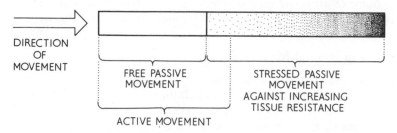

Fig. 14/1 Full stressed passive movement is greater than active movement and greater than free passive movement.

constitute prime movement, but which can be isolated when the joint is in an appropriate position. These isolated movements together with distraction of joint surfaces, we tend to call accessory movements. Important components of normal movement, therefore, are *accessory movement* and *accessory range*; Mennell (1964), uses the term 'joint play'. These can only be achieved by applying a degree of force, and are thus all stressed passive movements. This characteristic of accessory movement and their integrity is an important safeguard against the stresses of normal life.

Force in Abnormal Movement

Abnormality begins when either discomfort or resistance is greater than normal. The beginnings of the abnormal are to be noticed long before there is frank painful limitation of movement and are usually to be found in accessory movement before gross primary range is affected. For example:

1. Movement is full, but becomes uncomfortable earlier in the range than is normal

2. Movement is full, but the quality of the resistance is denser, or offered earlier in the range than in the normal

3. Movement is full, but an element of muscle spasm may be picked up by quick or careless handling.

The ability to distinguish between the resistance of tissue tension and that of muscle activity (be it active resistance or spasm) is one of the first things that the manipulator must acquire. These elements are subtle and difficult to learn, but their recognition forms the basis of informed and safe manipulation. An attempt has been made to illustrate them as Movement Diagrams (Hickling and Maitland, 1970).

It is in talking of this kind of phenomenon that manipulators are sometimes accused of mumbo-jumbo. Critics should be ready to accept that the manipulator may be attempting to convey acute perception with rather inadequate terminology. It is perhaps only fair to add that the manipulator should beware of self-deception about illusory or subjective data.

Amplitude/Force/Velocity

The word 'amplitude' is used to describe the size of a movement, and an important skill that the manipulator must acquire is to be able to perform a forceful, high velocity movement through a small amplitude.

The distinction between 'positioning' and 'execution' must be drawn here. Many manoeuvres are quite complex and involve considerable joint movement before the position is reached from which the manipulation is performed; insufficient care in the preliminary positioning leads to ineffective, dangerous, or unnecessarily painful manipulation.

To take a single example: the manipulator may wish to apply a high velocity thrust at the end of a generalised rotation of the trunk. During this, from position of rest to the end of the manipulation, the trunk may be seen to move through about 90° represented diagrammatically in Fig. 14/2. The major part of this movement is positioning, and only the last few degrees are manipulation proper.

Somewhere about point B. various things occur:

1. The manipulator encounters resistance and can only continue by using increased force to enter a stressed passive range.

2. The type of resistance has to be evaluated. Muscle activity (spasm or active resistance) must be distinguished from tissue tension, and the manoeuvre then modified or abandoned.

3. If the resistance is of an expected and acceptable kind, the

manipulator may use considerable force and velocity to overcome it, but must be able so to control matters that movement stops at the end of normal range at point C.

4. At the same time, the manipulator must be sure that any pain provoked is of an acceptable degree and position.

If muscle activity is not recognised, or uncontrolled force takes movement beyond normal range, either the joint is not moved effectively, or trauma occurs, or both.

The skilled manipulator may choose to move from resting position to the end of the manoeuvre in one continuous, large amplitude

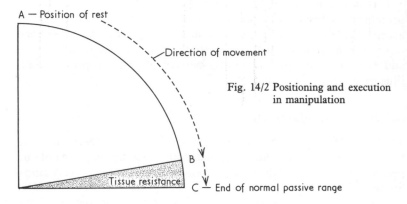

Fig. 14/2 Positioning and execution in manipulation

movement, combining positioning and execution. Novices must beware of copying this, for they cannot possibly have the necessary perception and control to make such movement accurate, effective and safe. Students should separate positioning from execution, and realise that skill in the first is more difficult than, and takes precedence over, skill in the second.

Mobilisation

The word 'mobilisation' has now acquired two distinct meanings.

1. The first meaning is of long-standing use in the orthopaedic sphere. Here, 'to mobilise' means to induce and encourage mobility by whatever means are suitable. It may range from giving a recumbent patient her first gentle walk down the ward, to chasing young men round a tough training circuit. The implication is to 'push on', to stretch the patient a bit, by whatever means seem appropriate. It thus indicates intention but does not define method.

2. In 1964 Maitland first stressed the view that the manipulator

does not always need forceful techniques, but should often use more gentle methods. More gentle techniques obviously have to be carried out for longer to achieve their effect, and Maitland perfected a method of oscillatory passive movement, which he divided into Grades in order to introduce an idea of 'dosage'. Readers are referred to his books for more detail on this subject.

Maitland used the word 'mobilisation' for these techniques, and it thus acquired a second technical meaning: oscillatory passive movement, with the implication of 'holding back' from more forceful techniques. It will be seen that this is quite different from the orthopaedic use of the word described above.

Doctor and physiotherapist may well misunderstand each other here if, for example, there is a prescription to 'mobilise' a patient with back pain. If either is uncertain what the other means by the use of this word, they are strongly advised to find out.

In the ensuing text 'mobilisation' is used in the orthopaedic sense, and Maitland techniques are called 'oscillatory mobilisation'.

Manipulation/Thrust Techniques/Grade V

Recently the word 'manipulation' on the conscious patient has increasingly been reserved to describe a small amplitude, high velocity, forceful passive movement, usually (but not always) at the end of range. It is almost always into a stressed passive range, and the resistance being overcome may be a combination of the normal and abnormal. With few exceptions, however, it does not include forcing muscle activity, and this is an important safety factor.

This kind of manoeuvre is also called a 'thrust technique', or a 'Grade V' (linking it with the other Grades of oscillatory mobilisation described by Maitland). After positioning, the final thrust may not be in the same direction as the positioning movement. Osteopathic techniques described by Stoddard (1962), which are aimed at moving the apophyseal joints, give ample examples of this.

The above definition of manipulation is a useful one. The reader should be aware however that the word has other, slightly different meanings in the literature on the subject. For example, Mennell (1964), writes of 'examination manipulation' and 'treatment manipulation', an interesting use of the word which emphasises the interlocking relationship of examination and technique in practice.

PATHOLOGY: PURPOSE OF MANIPULATION

As already suggested, those who advocate manipulation by no means agree about what it is for. It only requires a brief acquaintance with both its literature and its exponents to make it abundantly clear that they are at odds about the disorder which responds to this treatment.

To take the simplest example – a common syndrome which presents with unilateral pain in the lumbo-sacral region and asymmetrical limitation of movement may be variously ascribed to disorder of the intervertebral disc, the apophyseal joint or the sacro-iliac joint. The manipulating physiotherapist who sits in the middle of the argument receiving similar cases with different diagnoses is perhaps peculiarly well able to appreciate this problem.

Where doctors disagree it would be unwise for the physiotherapist to have no doubt, but uncertainty need not lead to inaction. Naturally, confidence in diagnosis is a great help, but in practice no treatment is controlled by it. The diagnosis merely helps select the treatment, which is then controlled by reference to the presenting symptoms and signs, and changes which occur in them. The less certain the diagnosis, the more meticulous must re-examination become. It is this meticulous re-examination which enables the manipulator to treat, for example, the syndrome described above in a perfectly safe, methodical and effective way, while preserving a speculative approach to the nature of the underlying problem. This calls for a certain detachment of mind, which some find worrying or unsatisfactory. However, if manipulating physiotherapists can acquire this they may find that they are able to contribute evidence when the diagnosis is unsure, since the response to certain techniques can be retrospectively enlightening.

The reader is reminded that this chapter is about the principles, *not* the practice, of manipulation. The manipulating physiotherapist is strongly advised to study all schools of thought, not only one, and to try to cultivate a dispassionate approach of the kind indicated above; an approach which may cumulatively throw light on what is now open to argument.

DISORDERS WHICH MAY RESPOND TO MANIPULATION

Disorders which may respond to manipulation are now divided very generally under two headings, mechanical derangement and contracture and adhesion.

Mechanical Derangement

Here there is limitation of movement due to joint derangement or internal derangement of some kind; under this heading can be put such conditions as disc lesions, displacement of cartilage, impacted loose bodies, and possibly the impaired mobility described by osteopaths.

The purpose of manipulating is to move something: either a displacement may be reduced, returning structures to normal position and function, or it may be shifted to a 'silent position' in which it no longer causes pain. Manipulation of this kind does not involve trying to force the most painful and limited range. It is similar to the task of freeing a bit of jammed machinery – one does not usually achieve success by forcing the block, but by disengagement and perceptive jiggling in some other direction. Because of this, manipulation for mechanical derangement often includes distraction of the joint, and always involves movement into a painless or minimally affected range first. It is commonly, though not always, entirely painless.

Often it is not certain what manoeuvre will resolve the block. The manipulator must re-examine frequently to determine whether to repeat a manipulation or to use another one, and continuous information is needed about the degree and position of any pain produced. The patient's co-operation in providing this kind of clinical information is essential, and anaesthesia is therefore not used.

Contracture and Adhesion

In such cases limitation of movement may be due to contracture or shortening of tissues spanning a joint; this may be due to trauma, disuse or immobilisation, or it may be secondary to some underlying pathology. In this category may also be placed the localised post-traumatic adhesion.

The purpose of manipulating here is to stretch out or rupture the constricting tissue, and the manipulator necessarily moves into a limited range to achieve this. The treatment cannot be painless, but must always remain within the tolerance of the patient and the condition itself (not always the same thing). Re-examination to determine the effects of treatment is usually carried out at the next attendance, since some treatment soreness is to be expected and may obscure immediate evaluation.

Manipulation of an adhesion is characterised by a quick, forceful, small amplitude movement. More generalised or capsular contracture requires longer, tougher handling, and 'mobilisation' is probably a better term for this than 'manipulation'.

Findings at Examination

Mechanical derangement is characterised by the non-capsular pattern
defined by Cyriax (1978). There may be other clues, such as sudden
onset, a history of recurrence, and alterations in the position of pain
and pattern of movement.

An adhesion mimics mechanical derangement in that it also
presents a non-capsular pattern. The history may help to clarify, in
that there will be no history of recurrence, or variation in pain and
movement, and the onset will lack the typical suddenness of internal
derangement. Additionally, the movements will be painful and
limited in a way which suggests that they are stretching, not pinching,
the source of the trouble.

Where contracture is due to arthritis or capsulitis, movement is lost
in the characteristic capsular pattern for that joint (Cyriax, 1978). The
value of recognising the classic capsular patterns in this context is that
they will help to take the disorder clearly out of the mechanical
derangement category, and thus simplify purpose in treatment.

At the spine, because of the difficulty of examining one joint at a
time, these distinctions become blurred. The capsular pattern for the
whole spine is a generalised, symmetrical loss of movement; asymmetrical pain and restriction can arguably be attributed to mechanical
derangement, localised adhesion or capsulitis of an apophyseal joint.

Where there is doubt about the nature of the disorder, the manipulator is reminded of the attitude of mind recommended at the beginning of this section, and must rely on scrupulous re-evaluation of
symptoms and signs, something which in any case is mandatory. It
must be remembered that, particularly at the spine, in addition to
articular symptoms and signs there may be involvement of other
structures such as the nervous system, the dura mater or the arterial
system. Such involvement may indicate important contra-indications,
or special precautions to be taken when manipulating.

Manipulation under Anaesthesia

This chapter is about manipulation of the conscious patient; mention
of manipulation under anaesthesia is therefore brief.

Conditions requiring such manipulation may be either mechanical
derangement (such as dislocation) or contracture. Anaesthesia is
required when:

1. The manipulator is clear about the nature and the force of the

manipulation needed, without relying on information that can only be provided by the conscious patient.

2. It has been decided to carry out a manoeuvre which will provoke too much pain and spasm for it to be performed kindly or effectively without anaesthesia.

DANGERS OF MANIPULATION

There are certain obvious contra-indications to manipulation, such as instability, fragility of bone or ligament, active inflammation or malignancy, where any use of force is likely to damage the structures being moved, or harmfully involve others. Examples of such conditions include rheumatoid arthritis, ankylosing spondylitis, cord or cauda equina involvement and vertebral artery involvement. This subject requires close study.

There are other situations in which the dangers of manipulation are less, but in which it is regarded with reserve, as likely to be of little help, or as more likely to exacerbate than improve. Examples in this category are the presence of distal root pain or neurological deficit. It is true that these are less responsive to manipulation, and the mechanism of spontaneous cure in disc lesions must be borne in mind. However, occasional good relief of pain can be achieved, and it is a pity to avoid all such cases. After the proper exclusion of absolute medical contra-indications, safety and effectiveness lie in a methodical and meticulous approach by the manipulator, in acute perceptiveness in handling joints, and in observation of the rules of safety set out below. It is not prescription that can make manipulation safe, but proper application and technique.

SAFETY AND EFFECTIVENESS IN MANIPULATION

The Hand

The hand must have authority, and be strong, comforting and perceptive. It receives indispensable information and is the medium for a continuous two-way process. The manipulator 'puts in' movement of precisely the kind intended, and simultaneously receives messages from the patient and the joint in the language of tissue resistance and muscle activity. This process is constant, and should be seen not only as part of technique but as continuous examination, which at any moment may modify the manipulator's intention and method.

Pain

The hand should pick up signals of pain long before the patient has any need to speak, but clear verbal communication with the patient about the degree and position of any pain provoked is essential, not only after manipulation, but during preliminary positioning.

Spasm

Never force spasm. There are exceptions to this, but the novice should beware of them.

Force and Amplitude

As force is increased, reduce amplitude. Movement through one degree is unlikely to do much harm, even if the manipulation is ill-chosen.

Examination and Recording

A general principle of all treatment is that re-examination is carried out at suitable intervals; on some occasions the proper intervals for such re-assessment will be longer than on others. Manipulation, especially manipulation for mechanical derangement, poses the necessity for frequent re-examination, since changes in symptoms and signs may occur immediately after a particular manoeuvre. Re-examination may be necessary several times in one treatment.

A meticulous and economical method of recording examination and technique is an integral part of the process. This cannot and must not be skipped. Only so, can one keep track of rapidly changing clinical patterns in many individual cases; only so can changes in technique be remembered and future moves planned.

This is not different in kind from other forms of physiotherapy. It is just that the speed with which changes occur in manipulation may telescope the process. Grieve (1977), suggests that the allocation of time in treatment should be 'about 90 per cent thinking and 10 per cent doing'; these are fair proportions, recognising that the 90 per cent includes recording and planning future moves. It should be added that though examination must be sufficient to elicit enough information to control the treatment, there is such a thing as over-examination. In acute cases the physiotherapist must select only the critical assessment factors and so minimise examination soreness. The art of examination and recording is to achieve a balance between gathering all that is essential and eliminating what is not required.

GENERAL POINTS ON TECHNIQUE

1. Body-weight and strength must be used to advantage, and those who are lightly built must recognise that there are some physiques which they cannot handle. Those who have the advantage of strength must remember what has been said about the control of force and sensitivity in handling; otherwise their advantage may be thrown away or, worse, become harmful.

2. Explanation to the patient about what to expect, and calm reassuring directives during manipulation help tremendously in achieving the relaxation required. 'Let your foot touch the ground' said at the right moment may release tension in leg and back, and enable one to move the spinal joint effectively.

3. An ideal in manipulation is to localise movement to the affected joint alone. This may be possible at peripheral joints, but poses problems at the spine.

a) Even if it is felt possible to localise spinal movement in this way, it is not always clear which joint should be moved (a point already discussed). Techniques developed for moving an apophyseal joint may not be perfect for moving a disc protrusion.

b) The need for leverage to increase force and the desire for localisation are sometimes at odds, and a choice has to be made between them.

A reasonable rule is to achieve as much localisation as possible, but to bear in mind the point made under (7) below.

4. A basic principle in manipulating mechanical derangement is to distract the joint surfaces during movement. In doing so one necessarily limits movement somewhat in other directions; again, a choice may have to be made here.

5. Satisfactory positioning must always be achieved before a manipulation is performed.

6. It is not forcing of movements under voluntary control that is required (if this were so most patients would cure themselves). The abnormality to be sought lies within those composite elements of joint movement which include accessory movement and accessory range. It is within this territory that manipulation has its job to do.

7. A few techniques really mastered and done well are worth a whole bag of esoteric manoeuvres under haphazard control. The repertoire of techniques in constant use by experts is remarkably similar and remarkably small. The experienced manipulator gradually learns that what does not respond to manipulation by one person often will not respond to another; where there is success after failure it

is commonly due to greater skill in performance than to a more complex manoeuvre.

DEFENDING THE LIMITATIONS OF MANIPULATION

The practice of manipulation suffers from the 'hey presto' effect, both in the eyes of the public and, sometimes, in the eyes of manipulators themselves. This phrase is used here to describe the instant, dramatic relief of pain and limitation of movement after one quick manoeuvre. This phenomenon is impressive to the patient, particularly if he has trailed round the medical and physiotherapy professions without relief, and finally found it outside the medical sphere.

The result of such an event is reputation. What the patient does not know, and what the successful manipulator sometimes seems to forget, is that this is by far from being the invariable effect of manipulation. If ten people with back pain are selected indiscriminately and all manipulated, the chances are that one will be put right immediately; the rest will respond more slowly, not at all, or be worse for the experience.

Another factor contributes towards the prestige of manipulation, which is that there is a group of people who have a sense of well-being, of release and increased mobility, after manipulation of a normal joint (these can be matched by others who will feel stiff and sore for a while).

These two aspects of manipulation unite to produce a fellowship with a profound fidelity to its manipulators, often in the cause of prophylactic treatment. Such prophylactic effects have not been proved, and continued manipulation after the restoration of normal movement may well be harmful. If patients seek it they should be clear that it is not of proven use, and should evaluate it in terms of whether any pleasant feeling given is worth the money paid for it.

The heart of the matter, perhaps, lies in selecting a manipulator who recognises that manipulation cannot help all conditions, and who shows as much readiness to stop this treatment as to begin it in the first instance.

REFERENCES

Cyriax, J. (1978). *Textbook of Orthopaedic Medicine*, Vol. 1, 7th edition. Baillière Tindall.
Grieve, G. P. (1977). *Mobilisation of the Spine*, 2nd edition. Henry Kimpton.
Hickling, J. and Maitland, G. D. (1970). 'Abnormalities in Passive Movement: Diagrammatic Representation.' *Physiotherapy*, **56**, 3.

Mennell, J. McM. (1964). *Joint Pain: Diagnosis and Treatment using Manipulative Techniques*, 2nd edition. Little, Brown and Co.
Stoddard, A. (1962). *Manual of Osteopathic Technique*. Hutchinson.

BIBLIOGRAPHY

Cyriax, J. (1977). *Textbook of Orthopaedic Medicine*, Vol. 2, 9th edition. Baillière Tindall.
Gray's Anatomy, 35th edition. Longman.
Hickling, J. (1963). 'A Defence of our Limitations.' *Physiotherapy*, **49**, 9.
Maitland, G. D. (1977). *Vertebral Manipulation*, 4th edition. Butterworths.
Maitland, G. D. (1977). *Peripheral Manipulation*, 2nd edition. Butterworths.
McConaill, M. A. and Basmajian, J. V. (1977). *Muscle and Movements: a basis for Human Kinesiology*. Krieger Publishing Co. New York.
See also the Bibliography at the end of Chapters 12 and 13.

ACKNOWLEDGEMENT

The author thanks Mrs. B. Lindfield, Dip.P.T., Dip. Teaching P.T., Dip. Phys. Anthrop., of the Department of Anatomy, St. Thomas' Hospital Medical School, London, for her help in the preparation of this chapter.

Chapter 15

Drug Treatment of Joint Disease

by A. G. MOWAT, M.B., F.R.C.P. (Ed.)

Since the cause of most rheumatic conditions remains unknown, specific drug treatment is only available for a few diseases. These include gout, for which suitable drugs exist, and also various forms of septic arthritis in which antibiotic therapy is very effective. Specific drug indications for many diseases are indicated in the text. However, for most diseases including the wide range of soft tissue problems previously discussed, a wide range of non-specific drugs can be employed, such treatment merely suppressing the symptoms and having little or no effect upon the course of the disease. It is important, therefore, to use such drugs with care and to ensure that the effects of treatment do not exceed the effects of the disease.

Rheumatoid arthritis is the disease which produces the greatest confusion over drug therapy. The very variable severity means that at one end of the spectrum many patients will require nothing more than an anti-inflammatory drug, while at the other end, a few patients will require potentially more toxic drugs which do appear to genuinely alter the course of the disease and improve the prognosis.

Patients with inflammatory joint disease complain of pain, stiffness, particularly in the mornings and after periods of inactivity, and of aching due to muscle spasm. Drug therapy should be directed towards the cause of these symptoms, inflammation. It is rarely necessary to give muscle relaxants and the following simple analgesics are rarely helpful alone.

All of the drugs to be described are suitable for use in children in suitable dosage.

ANALGESICS (paracetamol; codeine and dihydrocodeine; dextropropoxyphene; pentazocine; Diflunasil.)

Simple analgesics have traditionally been recommended for the treatment of degenerative arthritis, particularly as they avoid the upper gastro-intestinal side-effects so common with some of the non-steroidal anti-inflammatory agents (NSAA), but this view should be re-examined. Clinical signs of a mild inflammatory response are commonly found in patients with degenerative arthritis; the known association with pseudo-gout and other types of crystal arthritis and the clear inflammatory episodes in those with Heberden nodes have challenged the long held concept of 'wear and tear' as the principal or only pathogenic mechanism in the disease. Thus anti-inflammatory agents rather than analgesics are often the best drugs to use.

Many of the existing simple analgesics have a disappointing action in arthritis and the superior analgesic properties of a red placebo compared with standard drugs has been elegantly demonstrated. Pentazocine, although it has proved an excellent powerful analgesic in many fields and proved valuable in the rheumatological orthopaedic field in the relief of postoperative pain, has not proved to be especially useful or powerful in the treatment of joint pain. The natural history of joint disease means that stronger analgesics such as morphine and its derivatives have no place in the treatment, except, of course, when severe joint and bone pain is due to skeletal metastases.

Products containing dextropropoxyphene, particularly Distalgesic, are the most widely accepted and prescribed analgesics and this may be related to the undoubted stimulant effect noted by some patients.

A promising new analgesic, Diflunasil, a fluorinated salicylate, has recently been introduced. This drug has the advantage of twice daily dosage compared with the need for three to four hourly treatment with the other drugs.

In general, combinations of analgesic drugs, although widely marketed, have no advantage over full dosage of a single agent. Other drugs such as those with an added muscle relaxant or anti-depressant should be avoided even though such drugs may help the patient and the correct dose of each product prescribed.

MINOR NON-STEROIDAL ANTI-INFLAMMATORY AGENTS

Aspirin and related drugs have been the cornerstone of anti-rheumatic medication for 100 years. Many would continue to advocate their usage as the first drugs in all cases. However, this view is now outdated. The advent of a range of new drugs has allowed us to critically assess each patient's drug needs and to tailor a regime to suit these needs. The basic facts and principles to remember are that firstly, a very large number of patients with rheumatoid arthritis and

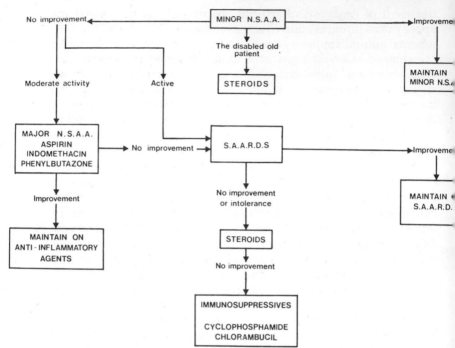

Fig. 15/1 Flow chart for the drug treatment of arthritis, particularly rheumatoid arthritis

related diseases have mild disease and will never require attendance at a hospital department, and that secondly, if drug therapy is to be instituted, it is sensible to move in planned stages from the least toxic, and in general least effective, to the most toxic and more effective agents (Fig. 15/1).

Many of these minor NSAA have been introduced recently and yet more will be launched shortly (Table I). They combine minor anti-inflammatory properties with a relative absence of side-effects, particularly those associated with the gastro-intestinal tract and are thus well tolerated by most patients. A response to treatment can be expected in one to two weeks.

It is important to appreciate, for reasons that are not understood, that patients show a very different response to drugs which are chemically closely related and thus a failure to respond to one drug in this group does not mean that all are useless. It is sensible to try full doses of three or four before proceeding to the use of stronger drugs. Careful comparative drug studies have failed to indicate a 'best buy' among these drugs and the choice of drugs will depend very much upon the

TABLE I   MINOR NON-STEROIDAL ANTI-INFLAMMATORY AGENTS

Anthranilic acids	mefanamic acid
	meclofenamic acid
Arylacetic acids	alclofenac
	diclofenac
Arylproprionic acids	fenoprofen
	flurbiprofen
	ibuprofen
	ketoprofen
	naproxen
Heteroarylacetic acids	tolmetin
	fenclozic acid
Indene acetic acid	sulindac
Enolic acids	azapropazone
	feprazone

general practitioner or rheumatologist's experience. In the short term these drugs do not alter the signs of inflammation in the patient, such as joint swelling, and even in the long term will only produce small changes in laboratory tests, such as the ESR. One is thus very dependent upon the patient's opinion of changes in pain and morning stiffness.

As with any drug, but particularly this group, it is important to ensure, before dismissing it as useless, that the patient has been given a full dose, that the patient has been taking the drug and that the patient is not trying to indicate other problems and worries when he describes continuing pain. A change of drug will solve none of these difficulties.

MAJOR NON-STEROIDAL ANTI-INFLAMMATORY AGENTS

The established agents, aspirin, indomethacin and phenylbutazone and related drugs are recognised as having major anti-inflammatory properties. It is likely that time will allow some of the newer drugs to be similarly categorised.

Aspirin

As already suggested there has been a swing away from the use of aspirin as the first line of treatment in inflammatory conditions.

The lowest dose of aspirin that has ever been shown to have an anti-inflammatory effect is 3·6g per day, while most patients will require 5 to 6g per day. At least one-third of patients will prove intolerant of such doses of aspirin within one month of starting treatment and this hardly seems the best way to gain their confidence at the start of perhaps 30 years of therapy. Aspirin and related drugs clearly have an important place in treatment (Fig. 15/1) and in recent years a wide range of aspirin-containing products has appeared, each attempting to overcome the most troublesome side-effect of dyspepsia. Few patients will tolerate large doses of soluble aspirin but dyspepsia may be reduced by the use of either enteric coated preparations (Nu-seal Aspirin), paracetamol coated tablets (Safapryn) and micro-encapsulated aspirin (Levius); unfortunately all of them are irregularly absorbed and hence have an unpredictable action; or antacid combinations (aloxiprin) and esters (benorylate and disalicylic acid) which are absorbed in this non-irritant form and then slowly de-esterfied often in a peripheral, non-hepatic site. These last preparations have the advantage of twice daily dosage and have a half-life which allows adequate control of night pain and morning stiffness.

Aspirin causes a wide range of side-effects apart from dyspepsia. Tinnitus, deafness, nausea and vomiting represent the effect of overdosage, whereas most of the other effects are not dose dependent. Many associate the indigestion caused by aspirin with peptic ulcer and gastric bleeding. There is little evidence that aspirin causes peptic ulceration but it may exacerbate the symptoms of pre-existing alteration. There is certainly a moderate increase in gastro-intestinal blood loss with aspirin but this is not associated with anaemia in most patients. However, a very small number of patients are hypersensitive to aspirin and in them the drug may produce massive gastro-intestinal bleeding.

Indomethacin

Indomethacin is favoured as the drug of treatment of night pain and morning stiffness. A large dose (50 to 100mg) taken at bedtime is remarkably effective in treating these symptoms, the drug enjoying a sustained action whether taken orally or by a suppository. The patient sleeps through the side-effects of headache, dizziness and confusion that can be associated with large daytime doses and the incidence of dyspepsia can be reduced, as with any of these drugs, by taking the capsules with milk or food. Use of the suppository has declined, partly because adjusted oral therapy is preferred, but more because it is often difficult to insert the suppository when there is significant upper limb and finger joint involvement; it is only available in 100mg strength, it may cause proctitis and it may cause dyspepsia by a systemic mechanism. However, some patients prefer suppository treatment and some of the new drugs are becoming available in this form for the control of night pain and morning stiffness.

For daytime use the initial dose should be 50 to 75mg in divided doses and the incidence of side-effects reduced by slowly increasing the dose at the rate of 25mg (one capsule) per week. The introduction of a slow release 75mg capsule may simplify the use of this drug.

Phenylbutazone

Phenylbutazone and related drugs are effective in oral doses of 300 to 400mg per day. However, to the usual side-effect of indigestion is added fluid retention and bone marrow suppression. Marrow damage may lead to serious reduction in the number of granulocytes and red cells and occasional blood tests and a careful watch for intercurrent infections are necessary. Because of fluid retention the drug should be used carefully in the elderly and in those with heart and renal disease. There is little need to use this toxic drug when there are so many safer alternatives available.

Following this type of programme the symptoms of a very large majority of patients with inflammatory disease of joints and soft tissue can be adequately controlled. It is important, however, that the patients understand the aim of treatment since those that expect complete relief of pain and stiffness will be disappointed. The commonest causes of ineffectiveness have been described while the temptation to change drugs too quickly or more especially to add a second drug to day or night time treatment should be resisted. Two different NSAA drugs should not be employed except when tackling the different problems of day and night therapy. There is no evidence that such drug combinations are more than simply additive in effect and indeed, the two drugs may interfere with each other.

SLOW-ACTING ANTI-RHEUMATIC DRUGS (SAARDS)

Patients with rheumatoid arthritis and occasionally those with other forms of chronic arthritis who are inadequately controlled on standard NSAA and particularly those with persistent synovitis and clear evidence of reversible joint disease, should be considered for treatment with more specific therapy and in general, this is probably the point at which the advice of a rheumatologist should be sought. An increasing number of slow-acting anti-rheumatic drugs (SAARDS) or treatments are available (Table II) and the therapeutic choice will depend partly upon the patient's circumstances and partly upon the physician's preference and experience. Once again there is no 'best buy' and at present it is impossible to predict which patients will respond to which drug. A significant clinical response will not be apparent for two or three months but is unlikely to be delayed beyond six months of treatment when a fresh therapeutic approach should be sought.

TABLE II SLOW-ACTING ANTI-RHEUMATIC DRUGS

Anti-malarials	Anti-lymphocytic serum
Gold Salts	Thoracic duct drainage
D-penicillamine	Transfer factor
Immuno-stimulants	Thymic humoral factor
Immunosuppressives	

Many of these drugs have been introduced into rheumatological practice on the basis of a known or probable action in animal studies or other human diseases and in many cases it is uncertain whether their success in rheumatoid arthritis is due to this or an entirely different action.

A clinical response will be associated with a fall in pain ratings, articular index (a score of the number of painful swollen joints) and morning stiffness and an improvement in functional tests. There will be an accompanying rise in haemoglobin values, a fall in the ESR, alterations in other acute phase proteins and immunoglobulins towards normal values and a fall in the titre of rheumatoid factor in the serum. In many patients there will be an improvement in the extra-articular features based upon vasculitis and nodules (see Chapter 6).

Simple oral treatment with *anti-malarials* has declined in popularity chiefly because of the rare but insidious, irreversible retinal damage. There is no agreement among ophthalmologists on the interval between eye examinations, although six monthly examinations are probably sensible, together with a month's withdrawal of the drug each year. Approximately 50 per cent of patients will show some improvement.

Gold salts and *D-penicillamine* probably act in a similar way based upon their chemical structure and type of side-effect. However, there is no cross-reactivity of side-effects and patients unresponsive to one drug may do excellently with the other. The commonly used schedules of treatment and the usual side-effects are listed in Table III. While there is good evidence that the clinical response or the incidence or severity of side-effects is related to the dosage of gold salts, a gradual introduction of D-penicillamine and careful tailoring of dosage is certainly associated with a lower incidence and severity of side-effects and allows more patients to be maintained on this therapy. The observation that the response rate to a second course of gold salts is lower than to the first has led to continuous therapy with the patient receiving 50mg maintenance intramuscular injections at approximately monthly intervals. This phenomenon has not been observed with D-penicillamine and this allows more flexibility in the drug's usage. Approximately 70 per cent of patients maintained on each treatment will show clinical benefit. With both drugs, monthly blood and urine testing is mandatory for the whole of the treatment period, since although side-effects become less frequent with time they remain serious and are largely reversible if treatment is withdrawn promptly.

TABLE III USE OF GOLD SALTS AND D-PENICILLAMINE

	Gold salts	D-penicillamine
Dosage and administration	Intra-muscular injection	Oral
	Test dose	250mg daily
	50mg weekly	
	Increase interval to monthly after clinical response	Increase by 250mg monthly to 1000mg/day
	Stop if no response after 4 months	Reduce dose after clinical response
		Stop if no response after 4 to 6 months
Side-effects	Rash	Rash
	Mouth ulceration	Loss of taste
	Bone marrow damage especially neutropenia	Thrombocytopenia
	Proteinuria → nephrosis	Proteinuria → nephrosis

Levamisole is the most promising of the immuno-stimulants, or perhaps more correctly immuno-restorants, the drug correcting to normal a wide range of humoral and cellular abnormalities in rheumatoid arthritis. The dosage of levamisole has not yet been established but it is possible that treatment on one or two days per week will be sufficient and be associated with a lower incidence of side-effects, particularly neutropenia or agranulocytosis and the 'flu-like illness' noted on the days the drug is taken.

Azathioprine remains the most popular of the immunosuppressives although there is little evidence of significant immuno-suppression and the exact mode of action of the drug is undetermined. Bone marrow damage and oral and gastro-intestinal ulceration are the common side-effects.

CORTICOSTEROIDS

Amid all the adverse publicity for corticosteroids their dramatic effect in rheumatoid arthritis has been almost forgotten. Perhaps this is as well as there are now few indications for the use of these agents and there are few advantages or increased safety with the use of long-acting depot injections or newer oral preparations over ACTH or pred-nisolone. With the wide range of NSAA available there is now little place for the use of night time corticosteroid in the relief of morning stiffness, while alternate day therapy has not proved particularly effective in this disease. A very small number of patients with life threatening disease will require these drugs but it is always worth trying to minimise or reduce the dosage by concurrent administration of a SAARD. Their usage (prednisolone 5 to 10mg/day) is perhaps justified in those elderly patients with an acute onset of disease in whom the prognosis is good and in whom complete drug withdrawal can be expected within one or two years. Finally, all are familiar with the patient who was started on high dose corticosteroids with insufficient reason many years ago at 'St. Elsewhere's'. Steroid reduc-tion under the cover of full doses of NSAA should be attempted but is rarely successful.

Side-effects of Corticosteroids

These include:

1. Peptic ulceration with dyspepsia, perforation and haemorrhage. The dyspepsia may be reduced by using enteric coated or soluble preparations.
2. Osteoporosis leading to vertebral collapse and bone fracture.
3. Salt retention with oedema, moonface and hypertension.
4. Liability to infection.
5. Skin thinning and bruising.

6. Muscle wasting.
7. Accelerated joint destruction particularly at the hip.
8. Inability to respond to stress since the normal hormonal balance of the pituitary – adrenal axis has been upset.

ANTI-DEPRESSANTS

Although any chronic disease can be expected to produce depression, the extent of the depression reflects the patient's understanding of the disease and the likely effects upon his employment, domestic and social life. Thus, anti-depressants are rarely required if the medical team has done its work properly. It is not considered that there is any particular psychological state (e.g. rheumatoid personality) either as a cause or effect of joint disease.

FUTURE DRUG PROSPECTS

Drug treatment of rheumatoid arthritis is currently most rewarding and offers the prospect of good symptomatic control for all patients and very real disease modification in many. Undoubtedly the use of SAARDs will continue to expand bringing with it the daunting prospect of ever increasing clinical loads unless the very close and responsible monitoring of these patients can be shared with general practitioners.

NSAA: Do we need further drugs of this type? Unfortunately the answer is yes, since each new agent will allow a further group of patients to be well-controlled with the minimum side-effects. Considerable scope remains for research into the modes of action of these agents (prostaglandin synthetase inhibition being only a small part of the story), into predicting patient preference, reducing the incidence of side-effects and simplifying dosage regimes.

SAARDS: More agents of this type will undoubtedly appear. It is to be hoped that increasing clinical experience will allow dosages to be altered so that clinical improvement is associated with a lower incidence of the usually serious side-effects. Further, it is to be hoped that research into the mode of action of these agents will lead not only to the development of predictive tests so that responders can be identified before subjecting patients to three or six months of potentially toxic therapy but also to lead to new information on the pathogenesis of the disease. Finally, better prognostic indicators for rheumatoid arthritis are badly needed so that those with the more aggressive and progressive disease who should be treated with

SAARDS early can be identified. There are promising signs that this may come from tissue typing.

LOCAL CORTICOSTEROID THERAPY

Local injections of a corticosteroid preparation into joints or surrounding soft tissues can be helpful in controlling inflammation. Such injections carry the risk of super-infection, a crystal reaction and bone necrosis, but these risks are minimised if a simple, clean, no-touch technique is employed and clear indications for their use are recognised. These include:

1. Intra-articular injections for the patient with one or two inflamed joints.
2. Tendinitis or tendon nodules, although the benefit with nodules may be transitory and surgical clearance eventually required.
3. Capsular and ligamentous involvement.
4. As a temporary measure in the treatment of median or other nerve compression syndromes.

Contra-indications

Contra-indications to the use of local corticosteroids include:

1. Uncertain diagnosis.
2. Proven or possible infection in the joint.
3. Severe joint damage, since they will be ineffective and may increase joint damage.
4. Severe local osteoporosis since this may be exaggerated.
5. A neurological deficit: because there is a risk of producing Charcot-type arthropathy (p. 101).

BIBLIOGRAPHY

Martindale: The Extra Pharmacopoeia, 27th edition. The Pharmaceutical Press.
Hopkins, S. J. (1977). *Principal Drugs*, 5th edition. Faber and Faber.

Chapter 16

Paediatric Physiotherapy – I

by B. KENNEDY, M.C.S.P.

In working with children the physiotherapist can expect a wide and varied case-load. The range includes neurological, respiratory, orthopaedic and rheumatic conditions as well as mental subnormality and multiple handicaps. That paediatrics has become a speciality of physiotherapy is due more to the differences between children and adults than to the actual conditions, some of which are specific to childhood, while others closely resemble the adult forms. It is the study of normal patterns of development, learning, behaviour and basic needs of childhood which provide the necessary framework on which to build up physical treatment for any particular condition. Observation of normal children of all ages will reveal a wealth of information which can be utilised when dealing with those less fortunate.

One natural advantage which the physiotherapist can put to good use is the child's enjoyment of movement. This is apparent from the earliest days when the baby learns to move his arms and legs, to play with his hands, and to kick off his blankets. It is seen in the toddler who is never still, and quite tireless in practising his new-found skill of walking. In the playground children can be seen running and jumping and twirling for no other purpose than the pleasure it gives them.

EARLY DEVELOPMENT

As the greatest changes in growth and development of the central nervous system, and therefore in the general activity of the child, take place in its first year of life, the study of this period is of the utmost importance. Probably for parents, the major milestones are smiling, sitting, standing, walking and talking. Between and around these achievements, there are a host of others – less spectacular but of equal or even greater importance in providing the total framework from which all activity springs. Physical and mental activity develop side by side, and up to a point are interdependent.

In early life, all movements are reflex. Later these reflexes are modified by 'higher', more complex ones, e.g. righting reflexes, balance reactions, and by willed movements. It is important to bear in mind the fact that the later willed or voluntary movements depend on the variety and quality of the earlier ones. Even the simplest voluntary movement depends on: i) an adequate stimulus; ii) the integration of the stimulus at conscious or unconscious levels and iii) the resulting motor response.

Interference for whatever reason with any of these functions will result not only in limiting the immediate response. Because the pathways are not working to their full capacity the sensory feedback will also be inaccurate, and there will be a deficiency of stored experience which, in its turn, will affect any future response. In this way, learning is affected.

Thus a baby who is backward in development may be so for a number of reasons.

LACK OF ADEQUATE STIMULATION

From their earliest days all babies need the comfort and stimulation of human contact. They need to be cuddled and to be fed in mother's arms, where they feel content and secure. They enjoy 'baby play' and quickly begin to learn about their immediate surroundings. Unfortunately, babies may be left alone for long periods, deprived of auditory or visual stimulus. These babies have no incentive to move and no opportunity to learn. Frequently the mothers of such children are depressed or may, from choice or necessity, leave their offspring with unsuitable daily minders. Sometimes, physically handicapped children, those who have prolonged hospitalisation or immobilisation are also in danger of being deprived, unless special care is taken to ensure that they have the opportunity to see and hear and touch those things which they would experience in normal circumstances.

LOSS OF SPECIAL SENSES

Blind or deaf babies will obviously be behind in activities requiring sight or hearing – though later they may partially compensate for this. There may be sensory loss in children with neuromotor defects, either because they cannot move, and therefore cannot appreciate movement, or because sensation itself is deficient.

BRAIN DAMAGE

Depending on the area affected, brain damage may result in impairment of the appreciation of sensation, of integration, or of the motor response.

MILESTONES OF DEVELOPMENT

It is more satisfactory to regard these rather as a related sequence than as isolated events which must be achieved in a certain number of weeks or months. Babies vary greatly and there is a wide age-span covering the rate at which a normal child develops. The following plan should be read only as a guide to the sequence of normal development:

1. Head control
2. Hands
3. Rolling
4. Sitting
5. Creeping, crawling and bottom shuffling
6. Standing and walking
7. Gait

These headings have been arranged to show the sequence in which the beginnings of control are acquired, but it is stressed that all these activities overlap and are related to one another.

Head Control

At birth the baby's head lolls when unsupported. If placed on his tummy he will turn his head to the side. In supine it is also generally turned to one side.

At six to eight weeks, when his eyes begin to focus, he starts to turn his head to look and will survey things in mid-line in the supine position. In the prone position he is beginning to lift his head off the bed.

At about three months he has full control of head rotation in supine, is getting good extension in prone, and is less wobbly when sitting on mother's knee. Quite soon he can lift his head in prone to look round from side to side.

By six to seven months he holds his head high in prone, and is beginning to raise it in supine. Although unable to maintain a sitting position, he can control his head if his trunk is supported.

With practice, head control and sitting balance improve. Head raising in supine develops together with increasing trunk and arm movements. Independent sitting and the ability to sit up from supine are both achieved by nine to ten months.

THE PULL TO SITTING TEST

This test is often used to demonstrate the degree of head control. The examiner takes hold of the baby's hands and pulls him into a sitting position (see Fig. 16/1). At birth and for a few weeks after, the head

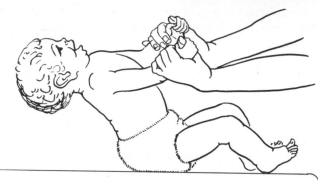

Fig. 16/1 The pull to sitting test – note the moderate head lag

falls back with no attempt to right itself. By three months there is less head lag and by five or six months it will compensate throughout the movement, and it may even actively flex as the child tries to sit up as soon as he grasps the examiner's fingers.

Hands

Hands are used for manipulation and support. At birth the baby shows predominant flexor tone throughout the body, and his hands are mainly fisted with the thumb held across the palm, though there is occasional extension of the fingers. By stretching the flexors of the fingers anything pressed into the palm elicits the grasp reflex, which in the first month or two is strong enough to lift the baby up by holding on to the examiner's fingers. The grasp reflex gradually fades in three to four months, and is replaced by voluntary grasping.

MANIPULATION

At four months, when eyes and head have gained some control, he is able to grab and hold a rattle and take it to his mouth for further investigation. Later he learns that it is fun to hold and release, to grab and throw. Also at about four months, he begins to play with his own hands, watching them move in front of his face. He also holds toys in his two hands, and transfers from one hand to the other at six to seven months. Early grasp is a simple flexion of the hand and fingers, the little and ring fingers playing the major part. This is known as palmar grasp.

By about nine months, the action of the hand has changed, the index finger has become the dominant feature, and is used for poking, and, with the thumb in a pincer grasp, to pick up quite tiny objects. This is the beginning of fine manipulation which will continue to develop over many more months as all the fingers become independent and fine skills are acquired by practice.

SUPPORT

Hands are used for support:
1. In prone, from about six months when the child pushes up on straight arms.
2. In sitting (see below and Fig. 16/3).
3. In saving reactions which begin to develop concurrently with the use of hand support (Figs. 16/2 and 16/3).

PARACHUTE REACTION

This test is often performed when screening children for cerebral palsy or other conditions where there is brain damage. The child is

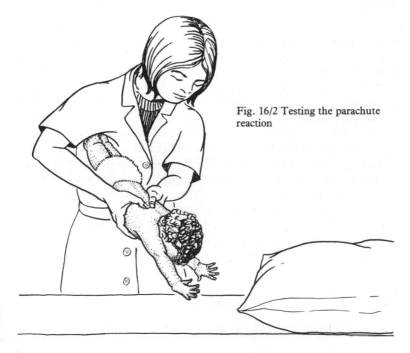

Fig. 16/2 Testing the parachute reaction

held under his chest, and moved rapidly forwards and downwards towards the bed – from six months onwards he should extend his arms and open his fingers as if to save himself – flexion or retraction of one or both arms indicate some neurological abnormality (Fig. 16/2).

Later still the child uses his hands to pull himself to standing and to hold on as he learns to walk.

Rolling

This is an important part of development requiring co-ordination of most parts of the body. The earliest rolling is from side to supine or side to prone, depending on which position the baby prefers. This in its turn may well depend on how the baby was nursed in his early days. Rolling from prone to supine occurs at about five months, i.e. when he can lift and rotate his head and upper trunk while the lower trunk and legs flex. Here is the beginning of trunk control and rotation. Rolling from supine to prone generally follows about one month later (head flexion in supine occurring later than head extension in prone), and about the same time as progress is being made in sitting.

Sitting

Before six months the baby can be placed in a sitting position but needs support. At about five months it is not uncommon for him to reject the position and throw himself backwards when his mother wants him to sit up. Active sitting starts at about six months, when he is able to lean forwards on his hands (Fig. 16/3(1)), but has no balance and is liable to fall. By seven months he can sit unsupported for one minute; by eight months he has acquired sufficient balance to sit steadily and to save himself with his hand if falling sideways. Between eight and ten months he is able to save himself if tipped backwards, extending his hands behind him (Fig. 16/3(4)). About this time he also learns to pivot on his bottom and to get from sitting to all fours. During this time, head and trunk control have improved in all positions and he is able to sit up from supine, rolling over on his elbow to do so, and at first pulling himself up with the other hand on the side of the cot. This pattern of sitting up, using trunk rotation, continues until the age of four or five years, when the child is able to sit up symmetrically.

Creeping, Crawling and Shuffling

These are all valid modes of progression of which a child may use each

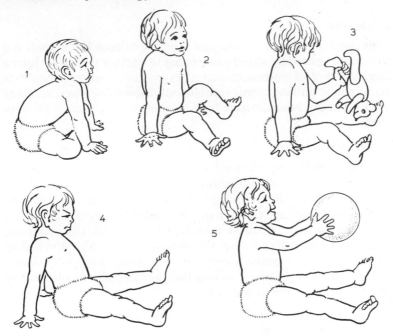

Fig. 16/3 This series shows the inter-related development of hand support and balance in sitting:

(1) Leaning forward on his hands at 6 months		
(2) Supporting himself in sitting	}	7 to 8 months
(3) Support with one hand while picking up a toy		
(4) Saving himself from falling backwards	}	8 to 10 months
(5) Balance and play!		

in turn, one only, or none at all. Unfortunately, there is great confusion about the terms creeping and crawling and in any discussion one must be quite sure that all concerned are using the same terms for the same actions. In this Section, creeping refers to progress in prone with tummy on the floor; crawling refers to progression on hands and knees, moving one arm and one leg alternately.

CREEPING

This may start with pivoting in a circle at about six months. Some babies push up on their extended arms and move backwards, others kick their legs and wriggle forwards. There are many variations and the preference for one is of little significance unless combined with other signs of abnormality, e.g. if a child consistently uses only his arms to creep and has difficulty in sitting one might suspect some neurological abnormality of the legs.

CRAWLING

This occurs at about the same time as sitting balance is acquired, and the child is generally already beginning to pull up to stand. Quite a large number of normal children never crawl, but go straight to standing and walking. Some crawl for only a few days, others for many weeks, but this seems to have little bearing on their general development.

BOTTOM SHUFFLING

This is a self-descriptive method of progress and is sometimes an alternative to crawling. Obviously, the pre-requirement is the ability to sit and balance while moving either one arm and leg, or both legs. Normal and abnormal children may be seen to bottom shuffle, so it is not a diagnostic sign unless associated with similar and consistent patterns in other activities, e.g. the refusal to use the other arm and leg and inability to sit symmetrically would lead one to suspect infantile hemiplegia. It is of interest to note that normal children who bottom shuffle are often late in walking.

Standing and Walking

Although the stepping reflex can be demonstrated in the newborn infant, this is only a transitory state which disappears in a week or so. However, at a few weeks he starts alternate kicking, and soon enjoys 'feeling his feet' when held upright with his feet on mother's knee.

By the time he is five months old, he sustains most of his weight, and starts to bounce. Most children start to pull themselves to standing soon after they have learnt to sit. They then enjoy standing at the cot rail; often their first steps are taken moving sideways along it. The actual age at which children stand and walk varies greatly. Some will stand at eight months and walk at ten, others not until eighteen or twenty months. The average is reckoned to be ten months for standing and thirteen months for walking unaided.

Gait

At first the child walks on a wide base in a rather square-set fashion. He has little balance and no movement of the pelvis. Gradually, with practice, his balance improves and his feet get closer together, and he learns to run. However, not until the age of three or four years does walking resemble adult gait, i.e. with pelvic rotation. Given the opportunity most children start climbing as soon as they get on their feet, but walking up- and downstairs using alternate legs is not achieved until two or three years, neither is the ability to stand on one leg, or jump on two. Hopping on one leg takes another year.

Conclusion

To summarise briefly, it may be seen that there is a definite link between the development of different motor skills. Rolling and sitting both require some head control; sitting also needs the support of the hands and arms; sitting up uses and consolidates the same pattern of movement as rolling and so on. It becomes evident that one must understand this progression of acquired skills in the normal child in order to appreciate and treat effectively the abnormal.

THE IMPORTANCE OF PLAY

The value of play to a child cannot be over-emphasised because this is how he learns. When a mother plays with her baby, he learns to watch her face, listen to her voice, to follow with his eyes, reach with his hand, to localise sound, later to imitate both sound and expression. He touches his mother's face and hair and finds it soft, holds his bottle or rattle, and discovers it is hard. So he learns about texture and

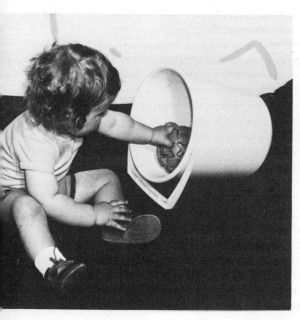

Plate 16/1 Playing with a plastic bucket!

temperature, shape and weight. Then he can learn about the purpose of things, rattles to shake, or punch, or roll, some noisy, some cuddly. He learns to select what is appropriate for his purpose – a soft toy to sleep with, a rattle to bang when he wakes.

Although good toys tend to be expensive, they are a good investment provided they are carefully selected. They may be supplemented by improvisations, using everyday household materials, such as a wooden spoon and saucepan which can be used for a variety of activities, cardboard boxes, particularly large ones, are great fun for climbing in and out and under, and later provide much imaginative play. A plastic bucket also has many uses, as container, seat, table, or just something to carry about (Plate 16/1).

While finding good toys may be relatively easy, what is more difficult is to provide the handicapped child with the right toy at the right time. Both age and ability must be considered as he will quickly tire of a toy which demands too little effort, and reject or become frustrated by one which demands too much. This is particularly difficult with those children whose intellect demands more than they are physically able to accomplish. The parents of such children are often grateful for advice at Christmas and birthdays, and this is often a good way to develop a wider concept of treatment. It is useful to be able to lend out the catalogues of the firms supplying well-made or educational toys, so that the rest of the family can see what has been suggested. Many local authorities have Toy Libraries, which help to provide variety and progression.

The physiotherapist will also want to give advice on the use and suitability of large toys, such as bouncers, swings, walkers and tricycles. It is, however, much more difficult to give advice once the article in question has been purchased; so it is essential to raise the question of these things at the earliest opportunity. In fact, this makes a good starting point to introduce ideas of management to parents when they first bring their child for treatment. It can be explained to them that baby may well be helped by one or other of these things, but that it would be better to delay buying any of them until his problems have been fully assessed. It is helpful to be able to try out the different types of equipment on the market, and see which is beneficial, and which harmful to each individual. Equipment should never be recommended for home use unless the physiotherapist has seen the child use it, and is certain that it will continue to be used to advantage.

Of this group of equipment, the baby bouncer is perhaps the most controversial problem, as everyone has a friend whose baby loves it, and for whom it works wonders! One must be rather wary of recommending these for handicapped children, particularly until one has made a careful assessment, e.g. it is tempting to 'bounce' the lethargic, floppy baby, but one must be sure that it is not in the process of developing extensor spasticity of the legs – which might be increased by the bouncing.

Care must also be taken when treating mentally subnormal children, though they may well benefit from using the bouncer to stimulate activity and build up their muscle tone which is often low. One of their characteristic problems is that of perseveration of movement, so strict limits should be imposed on the length of time spent in the bouncer. It is also important that other activities e.g. rolling, creeping and crawling which may be more useful developmentally, even if less convenient for the mothers, should not be neglected. The bouncer should be discarded when it has served its purpose, and the child is able to progress to a new activity.

Provided they are used with discretion and the contra-indications are recognised, bouncers can provide useful and enjoyable activity to meet specific needs. Occasionally the bouncer may have a more static use as an aid to standing or even sitting by giving trunk support to the very hypotonic child, to whom it is difficult to give the experience of an upright posture in any other way. It gives the physiotherapist a chance to position the child's legs and to encourage it to take some of its weight.

Baby walkers can be useful, but must also be used with discretion. There is a variety of these on the market, and each child must be assessed individually for his particular needs. This includes safety. If he is too tall for the model chosen, or too floppy, the child may cause the walker to overbalance. Care should also be taken where the floor is uneven. The older child may use the Cell Barnes walker, but should be supervised in case he tries to climb out and becomes stuck or falls.

Plate 16/2 Floor play using a crawler for mobility gives enjoyment while strengthening arm and back muscles

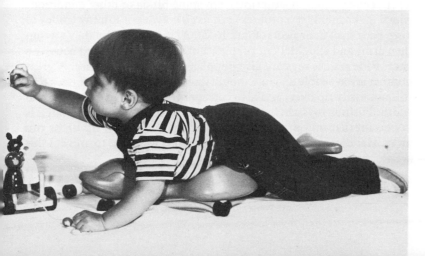

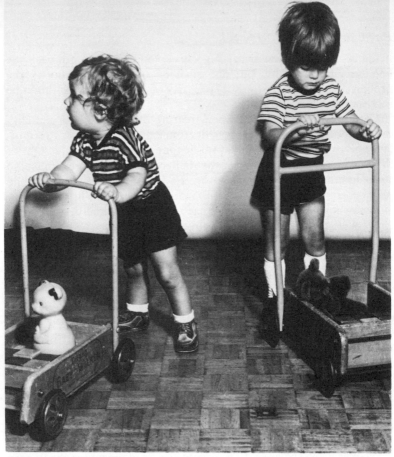

Plate 16/3 Pushing trucks may be a stage in learning to walk. Trucks must be the correct height for the child

Baby chairs and swings must be similarly considered for fit, safety and function. More will be said about these later.

It is important to remember that much early play takes place at floor level. Young children suffering from spina bifida or other conditions which make mobility a problem can use a crawler or tummy trolley to keep pace with their peers (Plate 16/2). At the same time they strengthen arms and shoulders in preparation for more advanced activities later. Ride astride toys are also popular and have many uses. A great number are available and one should look for the more stable ones that will not easily tip over, and also consider the variations of height and width. Pushing toys can help young children learning to walk, but it is important that they are of a suitable height and do not tip up or run away. Handles can be raised, trucks or prams weighted to prevent this (Plate 16/3).

Bicycles, tricycles and Go-karts provide exercise and mobility at some stages of treatment. If necessary, they can be adapted with seat backs and foot straps, and can sometimes be provided by the Department of Health and Social Security.

PHYSIOTHERAPY

Because their requirements are so different from adult patients, it is much more satisfactory for children to be treated away from the general department. Not only are the children helped by the more informal atmosphere and the presence of other children, but the parents are also more relaxed, and enjoy meeting each other and discussing their mutual problems.

At the first attendance, it is important to put both child and parents at ease before embarking on any particular techniques. Children hate to be rushed, and mothers are invariably upset if their offspring 'won't do what the lady says', or worse, stamp and scream! (probably because he expects either to be hurt, or left in hospital). One can learn a lot from talking to the mother, and father if he is present, hearing of their difficulties and fears, and what they think is the matter with their child. They are usually pleased to accept a simple explanation of the treatment and what it is hoped to achieve. Progress depends very much on co-operation between parents, child and physiotherapist and each needs to know from the outset what is expected from him or her. For babies and for the under-fives, work must be presented as play; even so, it is quite within their powers to understand that treatment time is purposeful.

A quiet and unhurried approach is essential for all young children, particularly for babies who easily become upset by sudden movements or noises. They in their turn can move very quickly, wriggling and rolling into dangerous situations unless precautions are taken to protect them. A baby must not be left in any place from which he can fall. In the ward, cot sides must be left raised and locked.

Powers of concentration vary, not only between one child and another, but in the same child from day to day. It is necessary to recognise the 'off' days and adjust the treatment accordingly, thus avoiding frustration and preserving a good working relationship for next time.

A few children in the under-five group will respond to a direct approach and can be taught straightforward exercises. Others need the incentive provided by toys and games for longer. At all stages it is important to maintain the child's interest and to change the activity before he becomes bored. Encouragement is the greatest spur; even a dull child will work for praise, whereas threats or bribes provide only another distraction. Praise, of course, must not be given indiscriminately, but it is usually possible to find some simple achievement to provide a starting point.

Games and toys must be chosen to provide the activity which is required and not merely for their own sake, otherwise valuable time will be wasted. Similarly, older children may enjoy the interest and companionship of classwork but it must be remembered that the aim is treatment of the individual and that each has his own specific needs.

In selecting a child for a class, various aspects must be considered; these include the age, personality and physical needs of the child, as well as the size and nature of the class and the experience of the physiotherapist. Most children begin to enjoy working together at about the age of four or five, but at this stage will need considerable individual help, either during or in addition to a group session. Classwork in its generally accepted sense is better delayed until the age of seven or eight.

Schoolchildren attending for specific exercises, e.g. breathing, posture, re-education after injuries, are generally more satisfactorily treated if their parents are not present. Once he has learnt them, the child is pleased to demonstrate the exercises to his parents and feels that he is responsible for his own treatment when it is continued at home.

Younger children, and severely handicapped older ones, are normally treated with mother present, so that she can learn what to encourage in his daily routine, and what to include in her home treatment sessions if these are recommended. Sometimes it is desirable to work entirely through the mother, so that it is she who handles the child throughout the treatment, the physiotherapist giving the instructions and explaining why they are necessary. This is particularly useful in the case of young children in hospital who need tipping, and can be persuaded to do so over mother's knee, possibly while the physiotherapist gives the same treatment to dolly or teddy.

Home Treatment

This must be kept as simple as possible, and within the limits of medical necessity, as short as possible. Parents and child should understand the importance of regular treatment, and over-enthusiastic parents restrained from insisting on prolonged sessions in the early stages which can result in exhaustion and frustration for all concerned. Notes should be kept of treatment given. Home programmes should be revised regularly so that they continue to be effective and the child does not become bored. It is also wise to ascertain that the treatment prescribed is practicable at home, e.g. that there is enough space to perform the exercises and that any apparatus required is available. Further reference to home treatment and management of the handicapped child is made in Chapter 18.

BIBLIOGRAPHY

Bobath, B. and Bobath, K. (1975). *Motor Development in the Different Types of Cerebral Palsy*. William Heinemann Medical Books.

Gesell, A. (1971). *The First Five Years of Life: A Guide to the Study of the Pre-School Child*. Methuen.

Griffiths, R. (1964). *The Abilities of Babies*. Hodder and Stoughton Educational.

Matterson, E. M. (1970). *Play with a Purpose for Under-Sevens*. Penguin Books.

Sheridan, M. (1975). *Children's Developmental Progress from Birth to Five Years: The Stycar Sequences*, 2nd edition. N.F.E.R. Publishing Company.

Sheridan, M. (1977). *Spontaneous Play in Early Childhood — Birth to Six Years*. N.F.E.R. Publishing Company.

A.B.C. of Toys, 5th edition. (1974) and other booklets from Noah's Ark Publications. Toy Libraries Association, London.

Chapter 17

Paediatric Physiotherapy – II

by B. KENNEDY, M.C.S.P.

CONGENITAL ABNORMALITIES

A congenital abnormality may be defined as a defect already present in the infant at the time of birth. Sometimes more than one abnormality may be present, for instance a congenital heart condition may be associated with talipes or congenital dislocation of the hip.

The three main causes of congenital abnormalities are: (i) genetic factors; (ii) intra-uterine pressure; (iii) intra-uterine infection.

The conditions described here are some of those most commonly seen in the physiotherapy department.

TALIPES EQUINOVARUS

As the name suggests, the foot is twisted downwards and inwards. The head of the talus is prominent on the dorsum of the foot, the medial border of which is concave. In severe cases the sole of the foot may face upwards and if untreated, the child walks on the dorsum of the foot. The majority of cases are bilateral (Plate 17/1).

Aetiology

The cause is uncertain, but there is often a genetic element. It has been suggested that the development of the foot is arrested before birth as a result of some unidentified infection of the mother, and that the initial abnormality may be in the bones with secondary changes in soft tissue. Alternatively, it is possible that moulding of the foot occurs when the fetus lies awkwardly in the uterus, and that the primary change is in soft tissue, the bones only becoming misshapen later, if the deformity is not corrected.

There are three components of the deformity:

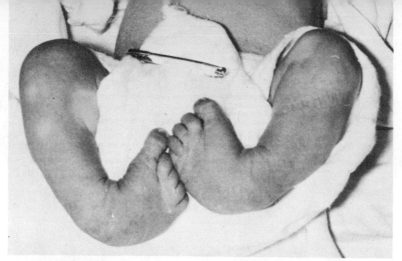

Plate 17/1 Congenital talipes equinovarus, showing severe bilateral deformity

(i) Plantar flexion at the ankle (equinus). The talus may lie almost vertically instead of in the horizontal position.

ii) Inversion at the sub-taloid and mid-tarsal joints. The calcaneus faces inwards (varus).

iii) Adduction of the forefoot at the tarsometatarsal joint. Some cases also have internal rotation of the tibia.

There is shortening of tibialis anterior and posterior, and the long and short flexors of the toes. The calf muscles are wasted and the tendo-calcaneus drawn over to the medial side of the heel.

Similarly, the ligaments and joint capsules on the medial side of the ankle and foot are tight and the plantar fascia forms a tight thickened band on the medial side of the sole. On the lateral side of the leg, the peronei and lateral ligaments and capsules are overstretched and weak.

Treatment

Treatment should be commenced early, on the first day of life if possible, and continued until the child walks. It consists of over-correction of the deformity by manipulation, and maintenance by splinting and active use of all the leg muscles, particularly the peronei. In severe cases open reduction of the deformity may be performed within a few weeks of birth as an alternative to manipulation.

If conservative treatment fails to correct the deformity operations to release or lengthen soft tissues on the postero-medial aspect of the ankle and foot are indicated initially, followed if necessary by bony procedures as the child gets older.

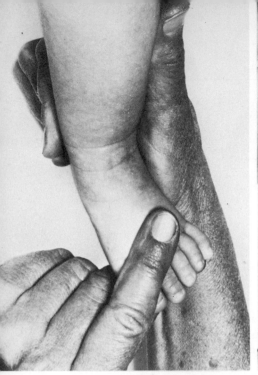
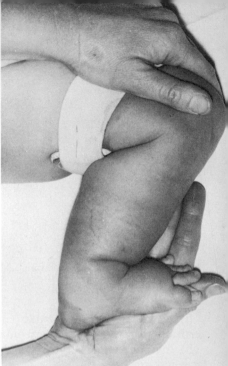

Plate 17/2 Manipulation to abduct forefoot   Plate 17/3 Manipulation to gain combined eversion and dorsiflexion

MANIPULATION

Manipulation to obtain over-correction may be performed on young babies by the doctor or physiotherapist without anaesthesia. In mild cases where no splinting is necessary, the mother is taught to manipulate the feet each time she changes the nappy.

During manipulation, the baby's knee is flexed and the lower leg firmly held to prevent any strain on the knee. Each part of the deformity is stretched separately.

The manipulations are:

i) To correct the heel: the heel is pulled down and out, stretching the tendo-calcaneus and structures on the medial side. For a good result the heel must be fully corrected in the first two or three weeks of life. After this time an inverted heel is unlikely to respond to manipulative measures.

ii) To abduct the forefoot: the baby's left heel rests in the palm of the physiotherapist's right hand so that her thumb supports the outer side of his leg, and her index and middle fingers hold his heel. The ball of the thumb acts as a fulcrum as the foot is bent sideways over it, the physiotherapist using her left thumb and index finger to grasp along the base of the toes (Plate 17/2).

iii) To combine eversion and dorsiflexion: the fully corrected foot can be pushed up and out so that the dorsum touches the outer side of the leg (Plate 17/3). Care must be taken to ensure that dorsiflexion occurs in the ankle joint and not in the sole of the foot. This depends on adequate correction of the tightness of the tendo-calcaneus; sometimes a tenotomy is needed to achieve this.

SPLINTING

Splinting may be by strapping, Denis Browne splints or plaster of Paris. The splints or plaster will be applied by the doctor and will maintain the feet in eversion and dorsiflexion. Strapping may be applied by the doctor or by the physiotherapist under his direction.

It is important that treatment should not be interrupted, so every effort must be made to maintain the skin in good condition. Three points are worth noting:

i) Care of the skin by painting it with Tinct. Benz. Co. before the strapping is applied. If, in spite of this, the skin becomes wet and soggy, gentian violet may be liberally applied and strapping continued. Occasionally it may be necessary to leave the skin exposed for 24 to 48 hours. Very rarely a baby may be allergic to zinc oxide strapping but may tolerate Dermicel or a similar preparation.

ii) Reinforcement of the corrective straps so as to prevent these from dragging on the skin.

iii) Padding pressure points with adhesive felt.

STRAPPING

This method of strapping to be described has been used by the author for many years and has proved satisfactory (Plate 17/4). Minor adaptations can be made to suit the individual case. The lateral malleolus is protected by a small piece of adhesive felt. Another piece 1 to 2·5cm ($\frac{1}{2}$ to 1in) wide depending on the size of the foot, is wrapped round the medial side of the big toe and under the base of the toes.

Three strips of 2·5cm (1in) wide zinc oxide strapping are used; one to correct each part of the deformity:

i) The first starts below the medial malleolus, passes under the heel, up the outer side of the leg and over the bent knee.

ii) The second starts above the medial malleolus and passes across the sole of the foot, around the forefoot (covering the felt). *N.B.* It is important that no tension is applied up to this point. The strap is then pulled upwards and outwards to the lateral side of the leg.

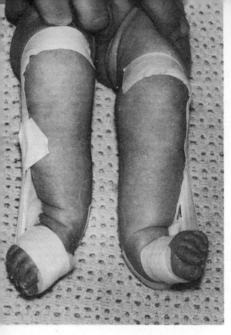

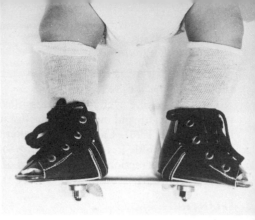

Plate 17/4 (*left*) Strapping for bilateral talipes equinovarus

Plate 17/5 (*above*) Denis Browne night boots

iii) The third strap maintains dorsiflexion and passes under the sole of the foot and up both sides of the lower leg.

Reinforcement by strips of zinc oxide 5 to 7·5cm (2 to 3in) in length, applied diagonally across the strapping on the lateral side help to prevent these from dragging on the skin. A cotton bandage secured with more strapping is useful protection and can be reapplied if it becomes soiled.

Initially strapping is renewed every two or three days until full over-correction can be maintained without undue circulatory disturbance, generally in two or three weeks if treatment is started early. It is then reapplied weekly or fortnightly. Some form of splinting must be retained until the child is standing when its own body weight acts as a corrective force. Before this time there is a strong tendency for the condition to relapse. In the later stages, Denis Browne night boots (Plate 17/5) may be worn during sleep times and removed for periods of activity. It is important that these should fit well and that the parents know how to apply them and are conscientious in doing so.

EXERCISE

Whatever form of splinting is used, the baby is encouraged to kick at first against his mother's hands, the end of the pram or, when he is old enough, against the floor. This strengthens his muscles and reinforces the correction of the deformity. Each time the strapping is removed, the peronei can be stimulated by stroking over the muscles, or along the outer border of the foot. After a few months, full-time splintage may be replaced by night boots (Plate 17/5), leaving the baby free to exercise during his waking hours, and the parents are taught to move the foot through its full range, to stimulate the peronei and encourage the child to stand.

Advice to Parents

Parents must understand:

i) The importance of continuous treatment.

ii) The danger of the feet relapsing if treatment is stopped too soon.

iii) The necessity of keeping splints or strapping dry. This should not be too difficult if the baby wears plastic pants.

iv) The importance of inspecting the toes to check the circulation, particularly after splinting has been renewed. The baby should return immediately to hospital if the toes become blue or swollen.

TALIPES CALCANEO-VALGUS

This is much less serious than the equinovarus deformity. It tends to recover spontaneously. The baby is born with the feet in a position of eversion and dorsiflexion. All the anterior tibial muscles are shortened together with the ligaments over the front of the ankle.

Causes

It is probable that the deformity develops shortly before birth due to the awkward position in which the fetus lies.

Treatment

Treatment consists of gentle stretching of the foot into plantar flexion and inversion, and encouraging active movements in the same direction. The mother is taught to do this several times a day. If the condition is severe or persists, a small splint may be made to keep the foot in plantar flexion and inversion.

CONGENITAL DISLOCATION OF THE HIP

Congenital dislocation of the hip (CDH) occurs more often in girls than boys. There are strong familial tendencies, cases occurring in siblings or in different generations of the family.

Dislocation may occur before or at birth, or, in the less severe congenital subluxation, when the child starts to walk. The acetabulum is shallow, its upper rim is deficient and the roof slopes upwards and backwards at a greater angle than normal. The neck of the femur may be inclined more forwards than normal, so that the head easily slips upwards and backwards out of the acetabulum. Flattening of the femoral head may occur later, from pressure against the ilium when the child begins to bear weight, or from avascular necrosis after forceful manipulation has replaced the head of the femur in the acetabulum. Fatty tissue may fill the shallow acetabulum, the capsule is stretched and may show hourglass con-

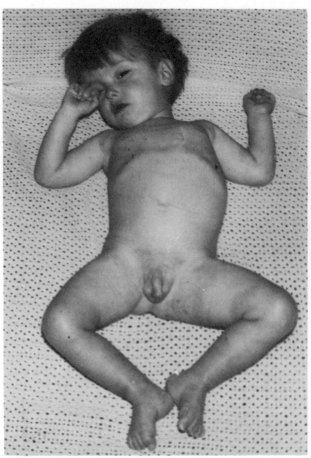

Plate 17/6 Asymmetry suggestive of subluxation of the right hip joint

striction, and the muscles become shortened in their abnormal position. Laxity of the ligaments may be a primary cause of dislocation.

Subluxation of the hip, which may proceed to dislocation, can occur after birth as the result of strong adductor spasm e.g. in hemiplegia or diplegia or to the unopposed pull of muscles in spina bifida. Regular checks should be made on children in whom hip abduction is limited (Plate 17/6).

Signs

The most significant signs are limitation of abduction of the flexed hip and shortening of the leg. With the baby's hip flexed to 90° it should be possible to abduct both hips so that the thighs are lying in the same plane. If the dislocation is bilateral the leg shortening may be less apparent though there is often some inequality and abduction is limited on both sides. There is also broadening of the perineum. Sometimes a click is obtained when moving the hips into the flexion abduction position, and this may be due to the head of the femur riding over the rim of the acetabulum, but clicks can also be elicited in normal joints. Diagnosis is confirmed by radiograph.

If the dislocation remains unreduced when the child starts to walk, the mechanical instability of the joint and loss of a fixed point of insertion for the abductors of the hip results in the inability of these muscles to hold the pelvis level when the patient stands on the affected leg (Trendelenburg's sign). Fortunately, this is rarely seen except in older patients. Testing for signs of dislocation of the hips is now part of the routine examination of neonates. Early diagnosis is important, as the prognosis is very much better if treatment is commenced soon after birth.

Treatment

In young babies, simple reduction may be performed without anaesthetic, and maintained by a Denis Browne, Barlow or Von Rosen splint, all of which are designed to keep the hips in flexion and abduction. These splints may also be used for babies whose hips are not dislocated but who have physical or radiological signs of subluxation, while for very mild cases in young babies, the use of double nappies may be sufficient to keep the hips abducted.

If it is not possible to obtain full abduction without the use of forceful manipulation, reduction may be obtained by: i) traction to both legs with gradually increasing abduction until the legs are at an angle of 180°; ii) adductor tenotomy followed by gentle manipulation

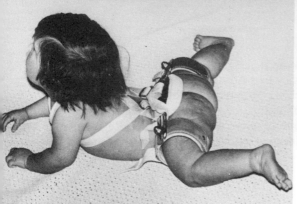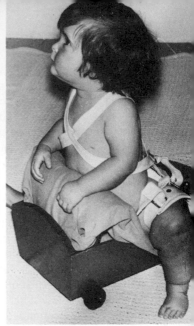

Plate 17/7 (a & b) Denis Browne splint for C. D. H.; this maintains hip abduction but allows child to move the rest of the body freely

or iii) open operation if all attempts at closed reduction have failed.

All three procedures are followed by plaster of Paris with the hips in 90°.flexion and 90° abduction (the frog position), or in any position in which the reduction is most stable.

Treatment lasts until the head of the femur has been maintained in the acetabulum for at least one year and the acetabular roof has formed satisfactorily. For the last few months plaster may be replaced by a Denis Browne splint (Plate 17/7a). This maintains the hip abduction but allows the child to move the rest of the body freely. At this stage the child is encouraged to move his legs by sitting astride a truck or other suitable toy and paddling himself along (Plate 17/7b). He can also learn to walk and climb in the splint. In this way the rotary movement at the hip joint drives the head of the femur into the acetabulum, so stimulating normal shape and growth.

Following removal of splinting, the child walks on a wide base but gradually the gait becomes normal without further treatment. Exercises to teach the child to walk on a narrow base are contra-indicated as strong adduction too early may cause re-dislocation.

TORTICOLLIS

Wry neck or torticollis is occasionally seen by the physiotherapist. The child holds his head tilted to one side so that the ear is drawn towards the shoulder on the tight side. At the same time, the face is turned to the opposite side.

Structural Torticollis

A cervical hemivertebra may be the cause of torticollis but this is very rare and there is no treatment.

Infantile Torticollis

This is the type most commonly seen. It is often associated with sternomastoid tumour. A small hard lump consisting of fibrous scar tissue can be felt in the muscle belly at birth or shortly afterwards. The scar tissue contracts, so shortening the muscle. The clavicular head of the muscle may stand out in a tight band and the head is pulled over into the typical position (Fig. 17/1).

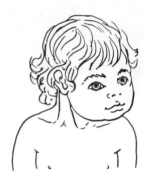

Fig. 17/1 Infantile torticollis showing the sternomastoid muscle

CAUSE

The cause is unknown. A fibrous tumour may be present before birth or a haematoma may result from a traction injury during birth. Facial asymmetry and moulding of the head is often a factor, but this slowly improves if the muscle can be stretched and the head held straight. In untreated cases facial asymmetry may persist and after some years it becomes irreversible.

Fetal Torticollis

The appearances are similar to the infantile type described above but there is no tumour and little or no limitation of passive movement.

Asymmetric moulding of the head, probably from the position in utero, results in it being held consistently on one side. Active rotation to the other side is made difficult by the shape of the head. The infant frequently prefers to lie on one side only.

The condition often improves spontaneously as the baby grows and gets more active. The moulding of the head disappears more slowly in about a year.

Physiotherapy is sometimes given if the infant is slow to start moving. It follows the pattern given below.

Treatment

Physiotherapy, consisting of stretching, active exercises and general management, should be started early, usually at about four weeks, and is generally successful up to the age of six months. After this time the muscle is more difficult to stretch, and although it is worth while

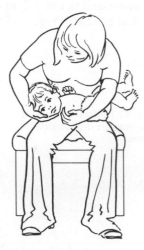

Fig. 17/2 Mother manipulating her child's torticollis

continuing with physiotherapy, tenotomy of the sterno-mastoid may have to be considered at a later date.

STRETCHING

The movements performed in stretching the sterno-mastoid are:

    i) Side flexion of the head and neck away from the tight side;

    ii) rotation of the head so that the face is turned towards the tight side;

    iii) both movements combined, side flexion followed by rotation.

If the baby is small the mother can do the stretching while he lies on her lap (Fig. 17/2). In order to make him feel secure, she must sit on a chair low enough for both feet to rest firmly on the floor. The baby lies across the mother's knee, in the case of a right torticollis his head rests on her right knee. She places her left hand over the point of his right shoulder to hold it down; her left forearm keeps his arms and trunk tucked close in to her own body. She places her right hand on the right side of the baby's head, avoiding his ear, and brings his chin to the mid-line before performing side flexion (bringing the head towards her) and rotation (turning the face away from her).

If the child is too big, a second person must be enlisted to help. The child lies supine on a flat firm surface – a thin sponge bathmat on a table is ideal as it will not slip. The assistant holds the baby's shoulder down, while the mother takes his head between her hands and performs the movements as before.

Each movement should be through the fullest range possible, performed five or six times at each session and repeated two or three times each day. Although the mother must be taught to stretch the neck as soon as possible, the physiotherapist must realise that she is bound to be frightened of doing so, especially as the baby is likely to cry. She should be reassured and gain confidence, by being allowed to practise getting her hands into the correct position without actually stretching. When she is able to do this easily she starts stretching the neck under supervision before doing so at home.

ACTIVE EXERCISE

From about 10 weeks old the baby can be encouraged to turn his head through the full range rotation by attracting his attention with a coloured toy or rattle. At first this is done in supine, later in prone, later still in sitting. It is important to move the rattle slowly, giving the infant time to fix his eyes on it and accommodate to the movement. By changing his position, by holding down one shoulder the movements of flexion, extension and side flexion may be encouraged in a similar fashion.

GENERAL MANAGEMENT

The baby should be encouraged to lie on alternate sides; frequently one side is less used than the other.

The cot or pram should be placed so that the baby is encouraged to look towards the tight side; toys should be hung on this side.

The baby should not be sat up too early or for too long; his head will drop to the tight side if his muscles are weak or tired.

Ocular Torticollis

Occasionally children of three or four are sent for treatment because they hold their head on one side. There is a full range of passive movement and the child is able to correct the head position actively with help, but resumes the torticollis position as soon as left alone.

The cause lies in weakness of one eye and physiotherapy should be delayed until this has received attention. Usually the head is held straight as soon as the eyes are treated.

SCOLIOSIS

This is such a vast and controversial subject that it is impossible in this context to give more than a brief outline.

Scoliosis is lateral deviation of the spine which, because of the normal antero-posterior curve, is always accompanied by rotation. The primary curve may vary in degree, extent and location and is usually progressive. Secondary or compensatory curves form above and below the primary one so that the child can maintain an upright position.

Rotation is most marked in the thoracic region. As the vertebral bodies rotate to the side of the convexity, the corresponding ribs are projected sharply backwards forming the typical hump on that side. This is matched by a bulge on the anterior aspect of the chest on the opposite side. Complications of progressive deformity include impairment of respiratory function and in very severe cases nerve root pressure.

True scoliosis, even when not progressive, is an irreversible condition and must not be confused with postural scoliosis, which is more often seen in physiotherapy departments and responds well to treatment.

Congenital Scoliosis

This is a structural deformity resulting from maldevelopment of one or more vertebrae (producing hemivertebrae). The ribs may also be malformed and be more or fewer than normal. There is adaptive shortening of muscle and connective tissue. Sometimes the deformity increases with growth, but although no improvement can be expected, the condition often remains static and symptom-free if there are good compensatory curves.

Paralytic Scoliosis

This may occur as a result of muscle imbalance and is a frequent complication in children with spina bifida as they get older, and also in many progressive neurological and muscle wasting diseases. Some cases of cerebral palsy, particularly the athetoid types who have an asymmetric distribution of spasm, may develop severe scoliotic deformities.

Treatment of the lower motor neurone types is on similar lines to that for idiopathic scoliosis. Those due to cerebral palsy must be considered in the light of their general treatment and management.

Idiopathic Scoliosis

Infantile idiopathic scoliosis may be noticed when the baby is two or three months old. The majority of cases effect a spontaneous recovery

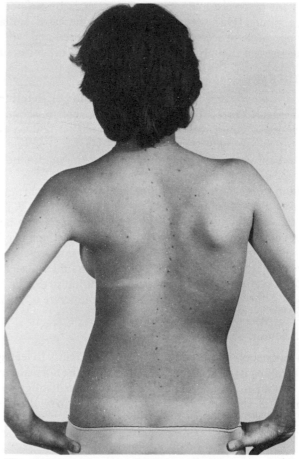

Plate 17/8 Early idiopathic adolescent scoliosis

in about a year; a few progress to severe deformity in spite of all forms of treatment.

Adolescent idiopathic scoliosis does not become apparent until the child is three or four years or even older and remains in a fairly mild form until the early teens, when rapid deterioration may take place (Plate 17/8).

Nothing is known of the cause in either case. Changes occur in bony and soft tissues as the condition advances.

TREATMENT

Mild cases which are not deteriorating must be observed regularly to make sure that the deformity is not increasing.

Treatment of severe and progressive cases is by supportive and corrective splints. If in spite of these the curve increases, spinal fusion or other operative procedures must be considered and will be performed at the age thought by the surgeon to be the most suitable.

PHYSIOTHERAPY

It is not possible to correct the existing deformity or to influence the progressive tendency of the primary curve. Exercises are sometimes recommended to improve the general condition and to maintain mobility in the secondary curves with a view to possible surgical correction later. Exercises may also be given in conjunction with a spinal brace or traction to reduce the deformity.

Attention to respiratory function is important, particularly in severe cases. Records of peak flow, forced vital capacity (F.V.C.) and forced expiratory volume (F.E.V.$_1$), may be made at the beginning and throughout the course of corrective treatment which may include surgery. The Bird ventilator is often used postoperatively to obtain better ventilation of the lungs. The child should be seen by the physiotherapist for several days prior to operation so that he becomes familiar with the respirator and is able to co-operate afterwards.

Postural Scoliosis

This is a much less serious condition, seen frequently in teenage girls. Strictly speaking it is not a true scoliosis as only the normal anatomical rotation accompanies side flexion, hence it can be distinguished from other forms of scoliosis by the fact that the curve disappears on traction or forward flexion of the spine.

CAUSES

The condition usually appears at a time of rapid growth. The child –

usually a girl – tends to adopt a consistent asymmetric stance and the general musculature is poor. One leg may be shorter than the other, causing the pelvis to drop on that side.

TREATMENT

More than an inch of leg shortening may be compensated by raising the heel and possibly the sole of the shoe. Gross shortening may require surgical intervention to obtain a better cosmetic appearance than a very high raised shoe.

Successful physiotherapy depends very largely on the patient's co-operation. As most patients are in the older age group, the initial explanation and planning of treatment to include only what is most effective is of even greater importance than usual. Attention should be paid not only to correction of posture in standing and walking, but also in sitting, with reference to school desks and chairs and whether she can see and hear adequately from her place in the classroom.

Correction of posture in front of a long mirror is useful particularly to start with, but this is not always available at home. Bilateral strengthening and balance exercises may be given to develop the feeling of a symmetric posture in movement. Home treatment should be kept to a minimum – one exercise done well is worth ten done in a hurry.

General health, including adequate diet, rest and exercise should not be overlooked.

BRACHIAL PALSIES

These are not very common but sometimes follow a difficult birth. They may be caused by pressure between neck and shoulder or by traction on the arm or head. There is damage to the nerves or nerve roots, resulting in paralysis of the muscles in the arm supplied by them. The prognosis will depend on the degree of damage. This can vary from mild bruising followed by recovery in a few weeks, to severe tearing of the nerves resulting in permanent paralysis and the danger of deformity. Fortunately the latter cases are rare.

Erb's Palsy

The fifth and sixth cervical nerve roots are damaged resulting in paralysis of deltoid, supraspinatus, infraspinatus, teres major, biceps and supinator.

SIGNS AND SYMPTOMS

The arm may be completely flaccid at birth but soon assumes the typical position of adduction and internal rotation at the shoulder, with pronation of the forearm and flexion of the wrist and fingers.

TREATMENT

This should be started as soon as possible with the aims of protecting the shoulder joint and preventing deformities.

A splint may be used to support the shoulder in abduction and lateral rotation, with the elbow at 90° flexion and the forearm supinated. Light splints made of Plastazote or Orthoplast are comfortable, and can be altered as the baby grows (Fig. 17/3(A)). Pinning the sleeve of the nightdress to the pillow is not recommended because of the danger of straining the shoulder joint if the baby moves.

Passive movements and the encouragement of whatever active movements are possible are started immediately and taught to the mother so that she can continue at home.

In severe cases, where splinting must be continued for several months it is important to see that the infant has opportunities for the activities normal for his age, e.g. in the prone position, rolling over, and sitting himself up, and it is essential to give the help necessary to achieve this.

The greatest recovery takes place in the first few months, after which time only slight improvement can be expected. Functional activities assume greater importance and the child should be given opportunities to develop the use of his arm and hand as fully as possible (Fig. 17/3(C.D.)).

Klumpke's Paralysis

The seventh and eighth cervical and first thoracic nerve roots are affected.

SIGNS AND SYMPTOMS

Paralysis of the extensors of the wrist and fingers results in the wrist being held in the flexed position. The small hand muscles are also affected.

TREATMENT

Small cock-up splints for the wrist can be made from plaster of Paris, Plastazote or Orthoplast.

Passive movements are started early and active use of the hand

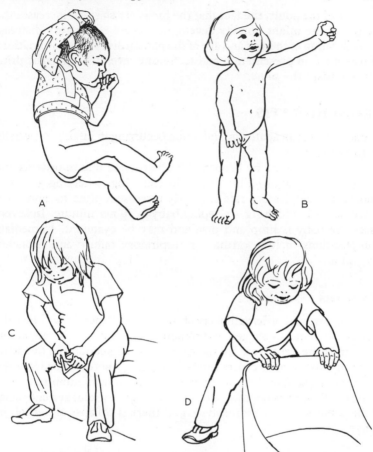

Fig. 17/3 Erb's palsy: A. showing the shoulder in a splint; B. showing typical deformity (right) – arm turned in and fingers flexed; drooping shoulder line and a disproportionately short upper arm; C. using toys so that the fingers of both hands are used; D. using both hands in pushing a chair

encouraged as recovery takes place. The use of two hands together should be assisted if necessary, at the appropriate age (six months), so that normal sensory development should not be lost.

RESPIRATORY CONDITIONS

These form a large part of the physiotherapist's work with children. Although the structure and function of the respiratory tract are similar to those of the adult, the fact that the lungs are so small increases the danger of the infant quickly developing severe respiratory distress. Consideration of the size and age of the patient also suggests variations of treatment in presentation and technique, even though basic principles remain the same.

BRONCHIOLITIS

Bronchiolitis is an acute viral infection occurring in infants, especially in their first year.

It is characterised by bronchiolar obstruction due to oedema and mucus accumulation. This results in coughing, wheezing and dyspnoea. The respiratory rate is greatly increased, often to more than twice normal, which for a sleeping baby is 30 per minute. In severe cases the baby is limp and pale and may be cyanosed. Immediate complications include cardiac or respiratory failure and bronchopneumonia.

Treatment

Nursing care and observation are of the utmost importance. The baby frequently requires oxygen and sometimes humidity. The upper airways must be kept clear by the careful use of suction. In the acute stage any disturbance causes further coughing, increased oedema and obstruction, so handling of the baby is kept to a minimum.

Physiotherapy is not indicated here. It may be useful at a later stage if the condition does not resolve e.g. if there is collapse of part of the lungs.

PNEUMONIA

Pneumonia is fairly common in childhood.

Bronchopneumonia

Bronchopneumonia is often preceded by an upper respiratory tract infection and may be a complication of infectious diseases such as measles and whooping cough.

Aspiration pneumonia follows inhalation of food or vomit.

SIGNS AND SYMPTOMS

Cough, fever and a raised respiratory rate are usually found.

Crepitations may be heard on listening to the chest.

A plug of mucus may block one of the smaller bronchi, resulting in collapse of the lung tissue beyond. This area of collapse can be seen on the radiograph.

Lobar Pneumonia

This is a more acute condition and results from bacterial infection, by the *Pneumococcus*.

SIGNS AND SYMPTOMS

There is a sharp rise in temperature accompanied by coughing, rapid shallow breathing and often pain in the chest. The chest pain is sometimes referred to the abdomen, simulating appendicitis. Consolidation of the whole or part of the lobe may follow the inflammatory reaction to infection. The consolidated area may be easily recognised on the chest radiograph.

Treatment of Pneumonia

In the acute stage the treatment is by drugs and, if necessary, the administration of oxygen.

In the sub-acute and chronic stages, where there is obstruction of the bronchi, collapse or consolidation, postural drainage with vibrations, percussion or breathing exercises as appropriate are given to assist expectoration and so clear the bronchial passages and to increase air entry.

Young babies may have to be treated in incubators or oxygen tents. If their condition permits, more effective treatment can be given if they are able to lie on a pillow on the physiotherapist's lap.

As already mentioned, mechanical suction should be available for use if necessary. The technique requires experience, skill and great care in order to avoid damaging the delicate membranes lining the respiratory passages.

In older children postural and mobility exercises may help to improve their general condition where this is poor following prolonged illness.

INHALATION OF A FOREIGN BODY

Inhalation of a foreign body is a common cause of collapse of lung tissue in children. One commonly inhaled object is a peanut, which because of its oily texture is not only difficult to shift, but causes irritation of the lung tissue. Other items include small beads, bits of

plastic toys, as well as teeth or fragments of tonsil following operation
for their removal.

SIGNS AND SYMPTOMS

These may follow a specific incident when the child was seen to choke
and cough. Alternatively, there may be no known history and the
symptoms are noticed over a period. The child may appear quite well,
but has a persistent cough and is often breathless on exertion. There
may be obvious diminution of movement on one side of the chest, and
a dull note on percussion indicating diminished air entry.

Radiographs are always a necessary part of diagnosis in chest conditions. In this case they will demonstrate the area of collapse and/or
indicate the position of the foreign body.

Treatment

Foreign bodies must be removed by bronchoscopy. Often no further
treatment is necessary. If the affected area does not re-expand spontaneously, physiotherapy may be given as for lobe collapse.

BRONCHIECTASIS

CAUSES

This chronic condition of dilatation of the smaller bronchi may follow
any prolonged or repeated chest infection, particularly if there has
been blocking of one of the larger bronchi by a plug of mucus or a
foreign body. A congenital weakness of the walls of the bronchi may
be a predisposing factor. The small bronchi become over-stretched by
the accumulation of secretions, which become thicker and more
infected. The elasticity of their walls is lost as well as the sensitivity of
the tissues lining them. Eventually the walls of the bronchi collapse,
forming cavities filled with thick sticky purulent material.

SIGNS AND SYMPTOMS

Bouts of coughing occur, often, but not always, producing purulent
sputum, greenish in colour and foul-smelling. These may be precipitated by a change of posture which causes the secretions in the lungs to
move into contact with healthy tissue and stimulate the cough reflex.
This is often apparent when the child goes to bed or when he wakes in
the morning.

In the long-standing cases there may be clubbing of the fingers and
even of the toes.

The child is often thin and small for his age.

Diagnosis is confirmed by a bronchogram which demonstrates the dilation of the bronchi.

Treatment

MEDICAL TREATMENT

This includes the control of infection by antibiotic drugs and investigation into the cause of the condition, e.g. the exclusion of cystic fibrosis.

SURGICAL TREATMENT

If the condition is limited to a well-defined area, lobectomy or partial lobectomy offers a good prognosis. The healthy remainder of the lung quickly expands to fill the space created by removal of the infected part and normal function is restored.

PHYSIOTHERAPY

The principal aim of treatment is drainage of the affected area. Therefore the physiotherapist must know the exact site of the lesion and the appropriate drainage positions. These are shown in Fig. 17/4.

Postural drainage, percussion, shaking and vibrations, and breathing exercises are used to facilitate coughing and expectoration. Sputum should be collected and measured each day. If there has been little or no sputum prior to treatment the amount may increase in the first day or two, but should then gradually decrease in quantity, becoming thinner, clearer and less purulent.

Some adaptations of treatment for babies are given on p. 274.

CYSTIC FIBROSIS

Cystic fibrosis is a disorder of the exocrine glands. The mucous secretions are abnormally viscid and tend to block the ducts of the glands, thus preventing the proper function of the organ as a whole. Lungs and pancreas are affected as well as the sweat glands, which secrete an excessive amount of salt.

CAUSE

The condition is inherited by an autosomal recessive gene, which if carried by both parents gives a one in four chance of a child being affected.

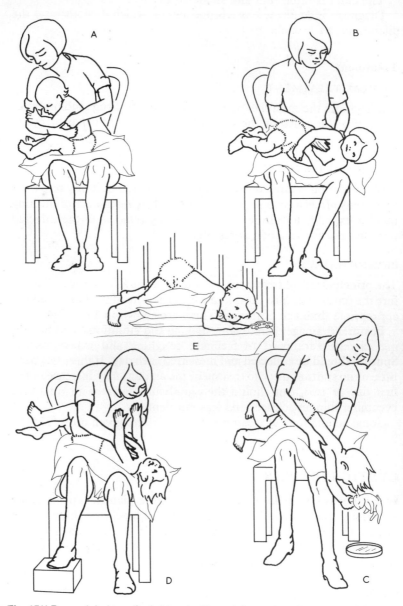

Fig. 17/4 Postural drainage for babies: A. Upper lobes, apices; B. Right middle lobe; C. Lower lobe, posterior segment; D. Lower lobe, anterior segment; E. Over pillows in cot – lower lobes, posterior segments

SIGNS AND SYMPTOMS

In its early months the baby may suffer from malabsorption, due to the lack of pancreatic secretions, and fail to thrive.

He is underweight and may pass a large number of pale, bulky and unpleasant smelling stools.

He is particularly prone to chest infections which do not resolve and frequently progress to a condition similar to bronchiectasis. Formerly these chest infections would prove fatal before the child reached his teens.

DIAGNOSIS

Diagnosis is made from analysis of sweat which contains an abnormally high proportion of chloride and sodium.

Treatment

Early diagnosis and treatment with the administration of pancreatin and other drugs, and attention to diet now makes the prognosis less gloomy. Particular care is needed to avoid respiratory infections and to provide immediate treatment when they do occur.

Chest physiotherapy plays a vital part and should be started in infancy. All areas of the lungs should be drained and coughing encouraged in order to clear the respiratory passages. This should become a daily routine at home, and increased to three or four times a day when there are signs of developing chest infection. It is therefore important to teach the parents to carry out the technique, and for older children to learn to perform their own postural drainage and breathing exercises.

ASTHMA

Asthma is a common condition characterised by spasmodic episodes of wheezing and breathlessness. Severe attacks may be prolonged and are known as 'status asthmaticus'.

CAUSE

Allergy is the most common cause. There may be sensitivity to the house dust mite, feathers, pollens, some foods and dust in the coats of animals. The house dust mite is a minute organism found in most normal situations but particularly in woollen blankets, carpets, etc.

In many cases there is a family history of asthma or hay fever. Acute attacks of asthma may be provoked by respiratory infection. A psychological factor is sometimes present; the degree of this varies in different individuals.

Irritation of the mucous membrane lining the smaller bronchi results in it becoming oedematous and therefore narrows the lumen of the bronchi. Further narrowing occurs from spasm of muscle in the walls of the bronchi. Air and secretions become trapped in the areas beyond the obstruction.

SIGNS AND SYMPTOMS

Some children appear normal between acute attacks, others have an almost permanent mild wheeze. Most asthmatics quickly become wheezy or breathless on exercise.

Acute attacks often occur at night or in the early morning. They may commence suddenly or build up slowly, with wheezing and a hard dry cough. The child feels unable to breathe and uses his accessory muscles of respiration to try to get more air into his lungs, but has difficulty in breathing out. The chest is held stiffly in the position of inspiration. Initially no permanent changes occur, the chest returning to normal between attacks. In time the lungs tend to remain hyper-inflated, the chest and shoulder girdle rigid.

Asthma and eczema are often found in the same patient, one deteriorating as the other improves. In severe cases appetite and general health are often poor. The child looks pale, small and under-weight but may be of high intelligence.

The degree of airway obstruction can be measured with a Wright's Peak Flow meter. Regular recording of the peak expiratory flow rate, (P.E.F.R.) may be used to assess the severity of the condition.

Treatment

Medical treatment can be divided into 1) that which is given during an acute attack and 2) long-term prophylaxis.

IN THE ACUTE PHASE

In an acute attack bronchodilators may be administered orally, intravenously or by inhalation. Salbutamol and aminophylline are the most commonly used. Ventolin (salbutamol) can be inhaled from an aerosol spray or nebuliser. If the attack is very severe or prolonged steroids may be given.

PROPHYLAXIS

Prophylactic treatment with Intal in a spinhaler is often successful in reducing the number of asthmatic attacks. Intal acts by reducing the sensitivity of the lungs, so it is important that it is used regularly, (usually three or four times a day) even though the child is well. Becotide, a locally acting steroid, from an aerosol may be used in a similar manner. Both aerosol and spinhaler require considerable skill and co-operation from the child and are therefore unsuitable for the very young.

OTHER ASPECTS OF MANAGEMENT

As many children are allergic to dust and feathers, bedding, pillows and furnishings should be of synthetic materials; these should be washed, shaken or vacuumed frequently. The child should not be in the room while bedmaking or dusting take place.

The child should be treated as normally as possible, attending school and partaking in whatever activities he can. Occasionally it may be necessary to impose restrictions on competitive sports or those requiring sustained physical effort.

Physiotherapy

In spite of recent advances in medical treatment physiotherapy continues to be of value in the following instances:

1. In the sub-acute phase of an attack, postural drainage and breathing exercises may assist in removing secretions from the lungs and encourage effective coughing. This is of particular importance when the attack has been exacerbated by respiratory infection.

2. Where complete control by medication is not being achieved, some children can be helped by learning relaxation, diaphragmatic breathing and general mobility exercises. This can help to minimise the development of the typical barrel chest deformity and posture. Mild wheezes can sometimes be controlled by positioning and relaxation; parents are more confident if they can help their children in this way and are able to institute postural drainage for those children prone to chest infections.

3. Instruction and supervision of the use of Intal or other inhalations may be undertaken by the physiotherapist in the informal and relaxed atmosphere of the department. The makers of Intal produce a whistle which fits onto the spinhaler. This makes a whistling sound when the child breathes in, and is helpful in gaining the interest and co-operation of some young children.

SUGGESTIONS FOR CHEST PHYSIOTHERAPY FOR BABIES AND YOUNG CHILDREN

Postural Drainage

This is most easily done with the baby lying on a pillow on the physiotherapist's lap (Fig. 17/4). The baby feels comfortable and secure and can lie in the prone, supine, side- or half-side-lying positions with additional support provided by the physiotherapist's hands on his chest. The physiotherapist should sit on a low chair so that she can regulate the degree of tip by moving her knees. In Fig. 17/4(d) she achieves this by having her right foot on a low platform; in Fig. 17/4(c) she produces the same effect by extending her left knee.

Thus, all areas of the lung can be drained with minimum disturbance. If possible, the baby should be positioned so that his face can be seen, so that his colour can be checked frequently. A toy unbreakable mirror can be useful if arranged so that the physiotherapist, and the baby, can see his reflection, particularly when draining the posterior segments of lower lobes. Other toys, mobiles, or musical boxes may also be arranged to hold the attention of toddlers who are often happier treated on the lap, but still tend to get restless. They can, of course, also be tipped over pillows and are often found afterwards administering the treatment they have received to their favourite doll or teddy.

Details of the correct drainage positions for each area of the lungs are shown in the diagrams.

'Exercises'

It is quite easy to give vibrations and shaking in time with the baby's natural expiration. Toddlers will often imitate sounds and may 'sing' Ah-Ah-Ah while their chests are clapped or vibrated. Laughing is good exercise and if not too ill, most babies enjoy being tickled and encouraged to use their arms, by grasping the physiotherapist's thumbs while she performs 'circles' or 'hugging and stretching'. They quickly learn to participate; and so help to maintain mobility of chest and shoulder girdle, which can become quite stiff even in very young children.

All children love bubbles and blowing them is often a good introduction to the very young as well as helping to overcome the fears of many slightly older children, who may be away from home for the first time and view any new face or treatment with apprehension. Bubble-blowing requires little effort and therefore does not cause tension in the muscles of the throat or chest – even if the child does not blow them he enjoys watching and will reach out to catch them and a great deal of activity can be stimulated in this way.

Fat, lethargic babies are sometimes 'chesty' and may benefit from a spell in the baby bouncer. The activity improves their general musculature as well as increasing the rate and depth of respiration.

Simple direct breathing exercises should be commenced as soon as it is possible to get the child's co-operation. This varies from about the age of two years to four or even five years. The easiest starting positions are side lying or supine with knees bent. The child's hands rest over his diaphragm and he feels his 'tummy get smaller as the air goes away' and larger as he fills up again with air. This can then be repeated with hands on the lower ribs.

BIBLIOGRAPHY

Batten, J. (1975). 'Cystic fibrosis in adolescents and adults.' *Physiotherapy*, **61**, 8.

Carter, C. O. (1975). 'Genetics and incidence of cystic fibrosis.' *Physiotherapy*, **61**, 8.

Ellis, R. W. B. and Mitchell, R. G. (1973). *Disease in Infancy and Childhood*, 7th edition. Churchill Livingstone.

Gaskell, D. (1977). 'Physiotherapy for adolescents and adults with cystic fibrosis.' *Physiotherapy*, **61**, 8.

Gaskell, D. (1979). *'Cystic Fibrosis'*. Chapter included in *Cash's Textbook of Chest, Heart and Vascular Disorders for Physiotherapists* (Ed. P. A. Downie), 2nd edition. Faber and Faber.

Gaskell, D. V. and Webber, B. A. (1977). *The Brompton Hospital Guide to Chest Physiotherapy*, 3rd edition. Blackwell Scientific Publications.

Hodge, G. J. (1975). 'Physiotherapy for children with cystic fibrosis.' *Physiotherapy*, **61**, 8.

Holzel, A. (1975). 'The quest for the basic defect in cystic fibrosis.' *Physiotherapy*, **61**, 8.

Jones, R. S. (1976). *Asthma in Children*. Edward Arnold.

Lloyd-Roberts, G. C. (1972). *Orthopaedics in Infancy and Childhood*. Butterworths.

McCrae, W. M. (1975). 'Emotional problems in cystic fibrosis.' *Physiotherapy*, 61, 8.

Mearns, M. B. (1975). 'Inhalation therapy in cystic fibrosis.' *Physiotherapy*, **61**, 8.

Norman, A. P. (1975). 'Medical management of cystic fibrosis.' *Physiotherapy*, **61**, 8.

Scrutton, D. and Gilbertson, M. P. (1975). *Physiotherapy in Paediatric Practice*. Butterworths.

Chapter 18

Handicapping Conditions in Paediatrics

by B. KENNEDY, M.C.S.P.

A handicap has been described as 'a disability which for a substantial period or permanently, retards, distorts or otherwise adversely affects normal growth, development or adjustment to life' (Younghusband et al., 1970).

Cystic fibrosis is a handicapping condition (p. 269) and so is juvenile rheumatoid arthritis (Still's disease) (p. 70).

Some congenital abnormalities e.g. congenital dislocation of the hip, come into this category if treatment has to continue over a long period. Other handicapping conditions are:

Cerebral palsy
Clumsy children
Spina bifida
Muscular dystrophy
Spinal muscular atrophy
Mental subnormality

The needs of all handicapped infants and children have much in common. Suggestions for their general management and treatment are given at the end of this chapter.

CEREBRAL PALSY

Cerebral palsy is a common but very complex condition, treatment of which is a speciality in its own right and is fully described by Sophie Levitt in *Neurology for Physiotherapists* (Ed. Cash, 1978). It is due to damage or maldevelopment of the brain before, during, or soon after, birth. There can be many reasons for this, including intra-uterine anoxia, birth asphyxia and prematurity; the initial cause is not always known.

Signs and Symptoms

It should be remembered that the lesion is irreversible and non-progressive; the manifestations of damage may change as the brain and nervous system mature. Quality and variety of movement are always affected. Balance may be poor and position sense is often defective. Young babies may have difficulty in sucking. Usually they are floppy (hypotonic) in infancy but very severe cases may be stiff (spastic or hypertonic) from the beginning. Later, floppy babies may develop either spasticity or athetosis, (involuntary movements). Ataxia, a disturbance of co-ordination, is occasionally seen, and is sometimes found in conjunction with hypotonia or with spasticity.

Deformities may result from unequal pull of spastic muscles; the most common deformities are equinus of the ankle, adduction/flexion of the hip (in severe cases this may proceed to subluxation and dislocation – see p. 255), and flexion of the knee. In the upper limb flexion of elbow, wrist and fingers with pronation of the forearm may become a fixed deformity.

Associated problems may include those of hearing, speech, vision, perception, intellectual impairment and fits.

The severity of the symptoms can vary from mild disability with little interference of normal activities to major handicap, where virtually no useful movement is possible.

Treatment

It is generally accepted that some advice or treatment should be given early and that parents should quickly become involved (see p. 286). The selection and extent of specialised treatment will depend on the age and condition of the child, resources of the family, and of the services available.

In brief the following points about the different methods of treatment are important:

a) The student is advised to acquire some practical experience and understanding of the condition before seeking deeper theoretical knowledge.

b) Many workers may be involved in the management of the cerebral palsied child, e.g. doctors, speech therapists, occupational therapists, teachers, nurses, and social workers as well as the physiotherapist and of course the parents. It is vital that there should be close liaison and frequent discussion between them.

c) It is characteristic of cerebral palsy that signs and symptoms can vary in different situations. Where spasticity or involuntary movements are present they are likely to be more marked when the child is excited, tired or self-conscious. Treatment must be adapted to the child as he is at the moment, not the child to the treatment.

d) It follows that keen observation and continual assessment are an essential basis for treatment.

e) With experience the physiotherapist may learn to foresee and sometimes forestall future problems.

THE CLUMSY CHILD

In recent years a new category of handicap has become recognised. Compared to other groups of physically handicapped, 'clumsy children' may appear at first to have little to worry them; but compared to normal children they can be greatly disadvantaged and unhappy.

These children lag markedly behind their peers in physical activities and in school may make slow progress in learning to read or write. The latter problems are not related to intelligence, which may be of any range; they are due to difficulties of perception.

Signs and Symptoms

Diagnosis is unlikely before school age because of the wide variation of normal in the pre-school child.

Neurological signs may not be present although a few children with minor degrees of cerebral palsy may in addition have the same type of perceptual problems.

Children may be referred to the physiotherapist because of the following:

Poor balance
Frequent falls
Poor posture and general 'weakness'
Difficulties going up/down stairs
Clumsy hands and fingers

These children may find it difficult or be unable to:

Kick or catch a ball
Dress themselves, especially putting on pants or trousers
Manage buttons and laces
Manipulate a pencil, etc.

In school, problems may arise in copying shapes or designs (therefore in learning to write), recognising shapes (learning to read), copying positions or movements (in P.E.) or distinguishing left from right.

The child may be labelled lazy, inattentive, easily distracted or stupid. In fact, the child may try hard to please and become frustrated by repeated failure and if not recognised this may lead to behaviour problems.

Further investigation may show that body image and body awareness are poor and this may include:

1. difficulties in finger recognition
2. difficulties in coordinating both sides of the body
3. difficulties of balance reactions, particularly if sight is excluded
4. difficulty in judging distance and direction

Treatment

A number of paediatric units have pioneered treatment for these children. The results have been encouraging.

The treatment programme combines sensory stimulation, body awareness, balance and perceptual training. In some units this is planned by the physiotherapists and occupational therapists working closely together; the occupational therapists undertake perceptual training, the physiotherapists the motor development.

The child's difficulties should be discussed with him so that he can understand the reasons for treatment. If the parents are present during the initial investigations, they too will be able to see where the problems lie. Careful explanation as to how help may be given may relieve tension and pressure on the child both from school and home routine. Allowing a little extra time may enable the child to become more independent and less frustrated. Dressing can be made easier, by using Velcro fastening, until the child becomes more skilful in managing buttons and laces; elastic at the waist of shorts or skirt, or slip-on shoes. Games can be adapted so that the child is able to participate at his own level, or to help to develop or practise new skills.

SPINA BIFIDA

A more detailed account of this condition is given by Olwen Nettles in *Neurology for Physiotherapists* (Ed. Cash, 1978). As it is one of the commonest physical handicaps at present found in children of school age, some of the basic points are also included here.

Maldevelopment of the vertebrae and spinal cord may occur at any level but is most frequent in the lower dorsal or lumbar region. The cause is unknown but there may be a genetic element.

Signs and Symptoms

Involvement of the spinal cord in the swelling (myelocele or mening-omyelocele) which protrudes through the open arch of the vertebrae produces a mainly flaccid paralysis below the level of the lesion, though some spasticity may also be present. In addition there is severe sensory loss, the implications of which must be continually borne in mind. The greatest care must be taken when moving on rough surfaces or near heaters (radiators) as well as seeing that clothing, calipers or toys do not cause friction or undue pressure.

The degree of involvement of the lower trunk and legs depends on the level and severity of the lesion. In high lesions the whole trunk and upper limbs may be affected to some degree.

COMPLICATIONS

1) Hydrocephalus is frequently present and it appears soon after birth. If a valve has been inserted there is the possibility of it becoming blocked. Physiotherapists and parents should be aware of this and report signs of drowsiness or vomiting to the doctor or surgeon at once.

2) Deformities may be present at birth or may occur later if muscle tension is not balanced. Unopposed flexors and adductors of the hip joint quite often cause subluxation or dislocation of this joint.

3) Urinary incontinence predisposes to skin inflammation and chronic urinary infection; absence of bowel control is a major problem – (but the danger of infection is absent).

4) Fractures are liable to occur particularly following immobilisation in plaster. Where possible weight-bearing and full activity should be encouraged so as to maintain, as far as possible, the circulation and stimulation of bone growth.

Treatment

Early management is again important and is directed towards giving maximum normal experience, developing what muscle potential is available and obtaining independent mobility as soon as possible. If the child's condition permits, calipers for walking may be fitted between the ages of one and two years. The motivation to get about unaided is strong at this age. Unfortunately this is not always possible and in any case achievement comes slowly, so it may be desirable to keep alive the spark of independence, by using some other means of mobility, e.g. the Shasbah trolley or a junior wheelchair. Various aids are available for walking. When possible walking exercises should be objective, i.e. the child should learn to walk as a means of getting from place to place, not merely as an exercise performed only in the physiotherapy department.

MUSCULAR DYSTROPHY

Duchenne muscular dystrophy is the commonest and most severe type. The muscle fibres degenerate and are replaced by fatty and fibrous tissue.

Cause

This is a genetic disease affecting only males but carried and transmitted by females.

Signs and Symptoms

Diagnosis is usually made between the ages of one and five years. Sometimes the child has always appeared floppy and has walked late. Walking becomes unsteady and the child has difficulty in rising from the floor; in order to stand upright he 'walks his hands up his legs' to compensate for weak extensors of hips and knees. For the same reason he has difficulty in going up or down stairs. The calf muscles may appear enlarged and feel hard, because of the fibrous tissue.
  Diagnosis is confirmed by:

1. Analysis of serum enzymes. A high level of creatine phosphokinase is present in muscular dystrophy
2. Muscle biopsy
3. Electromyography

  Between the age of eight and twelve years walking becomes impossible. Eventually involvement of the respiratory muscles leads to frequent infections, one of which is likely to prove fatal between the ages of 15 and 25.

DEFORMITIES

There is an early tendency for the tendo Achilles and hip flexors to shorten. When confined to a wheelchair knee flexion deformities are likely unless measures are taken to prevent them. Also about this time severe scoliosis is a frequent complication.

Treatment

There is no medical treatment which can reverse the inevitable course. The boy should be encouraged to remain active as long as possible. Reasonable care should be taken to prevent deformities of feet and knees, either by daily stretching or occasionally by night splints.

Scoliosis poses a bigger problem and a light-weight supporting jacket may be fitted at the time when the child becomes chairbound. Breathing exercises may help to maintain respiratory function at its most efficient level for as long as possible. Postural drainage may also be taught to parents for home use during chest infections. The provision of a well-fitting powered wheelchair and other aids to mobility are important.

Any adaptations to facilitate games and recreative pursuits obviously add much to the quality of life as upper limb weakness increases.

Other types of muscular dystrophy such as limb girdle dystrophy, facio-scapular humeral dystrophy rarely present in childhood.

SPINAL MUSCULAR ATROPHY

This is a genetic condition which can affect girls or boys. The most severe form is often known as Werdnig Hoffman disease. Floppiness may be apparent from birth or may appear in a few weeks or months.

Weakness is most marked in the legs and in the respiratory muscles. Active movement is only minimal though the baby may respond to stimulation by laughing and moving his hands. Usually the child succumbs to a respiratory infection within a year or two.

In the less severe forms the weakness has the same pattern of distribution but may remain static or progress slowly. Function can be improved and the child survive to adolescence or adulthood. A few mild cases are able to walk; some learn to do so with calipers and crutches.

COMPLICATIONS

1. The development of deformities, particularly of scoliosis and sometimes deformities of feet and legs.
2. Respiratory infections are always a danger because of the shallowness of breathing and inadequate coughing.

Treatment

Physiotherapy is important in the following ways:

1. To prevent deformities by the use of passive stretchings. The use and care of splints is important if these are appropriate.
2. Mobility should be encouraged, progressing to walking where the condition makes this possible.
3. Breathing exercises may improve respiratory function and reduce the risk from infections. Postural drainage should be taught to parents for use when necessary.

MENTAL HANDICAP

Many children who are eventually classed mentally subnormal also have slow and inadequate motor development. They may have poor musculature and balance and they may lack normal facility and variety of movement. Some also have specific physical handicaps associated with brain damage, e.g. cerebral palsy, sensory defects or optic atrophy.

Two categories of subnormality are recognised, a) educationally subnormal – mild (E.S.N.(M.)) and b) educationally subnormal – severe (E.S.N.(S.)). Educational authorities are bound to provide school facilities for all E.S.N. children of school age. In a school for E.S.N.(M.), the child of limited intelligence but unable to benefit from normal schooling, can receive some education. Many can learn to read and write and acquire some degree of independence. The severely E.S.N. child is unable to co-operate in any formal education, but some may be trained to a moderate degree of self-care and to perform simple tasks. They will always need constant supervision and help, and eventually it will be necessary for most of such children to have institutional care.

Because no other provision is made for them, a third group of children are frequently found in severely subnormal schools. These are the multiply handicapped whose combination of mental, physical and social difficulties make both management and training appear a formidable task. This is one which nevertheless can sometimes have surprising rewards.

Causes

Mental subnormality may result from cerebral malformation, injury or degenerative disease. Some conditions are genetically determined, others may be due to maternal infections during critical periods of pregnancy. There is sometimes a familial link but often no known cause is discovered.

MICROCEPHALY

The brain is small and lacks the normal number of convolutions. Although the face grows to normal size the skull barely grows after birth and the head circumference rarely exceeds seventeen inches. The child is nearly always severely mentally subnormal and in addition often has motor disabilities. Sometimes there is a familial tendency; there may also be a connection with infections during pregnancy.

HYDROCEPHALUS

There is increased pressure in the ventricles due to an excess of cerebrospinal fluid. The condition may be present at birth or occur spontaneously later; it is also frequently associated with spina bifida. Treatment by the insertion of a Spitz-Holter or Pudenz valve is sometimes successful in stabilising the condition; but unless performed early some brain cells will remain permanently damaged. In untreated cases the head grows very large to accommodate the increased fluid, thus adding to the physical problems of management and training.

DOWN'S SYNDROME (MONGOLISM)

This is the commonest identified cause of severe subnormality. The defect is due to an extra chromosome which increases the normal number of 46 to 47. The child is often the youngest of several and there are seldom more than one in the same family. Mongols are easily recognised at birth by their typical facial appearance, broad and flattened with small nose and slanting eyes; the tongue may appear too large for the rather small mouth. Hands and feet are broad and short; frequently the terminal phalanx of the little finger is in-curved and a single deep crease runs right across the palm (Simian crease).

There is generalised hypotonia with hypermobility of the joints. Milestones are always delayed and speech may remain infantile and difficult to understand. A large number suffer from congenital heart defects and a high proportion of these do not survive early childhood; usually they succumb to repeated respiratory infections. In general they are happy, sociable children, fond of music and anxious to join in all that goes on. The brightest can be trained to do easy repetitive work.

Metabolic Disorders

CRETINISM

This is the result of under-secretion of the thyroid gland and may be diagnosed at a few weeks of age. Although the baby appears normal at birth it quickly becomes dull, listless and unresponsive; the skin feels cold and is coarse and dry, the complexion sallow and the lips thickened. Without early treatment subnormality occurs, as the brain needs adequate amounts of thyroid hormone to develop normally.

PHENYLKETONURIA

This is a condition of defective amino-acid metabolism. It can be diagnosed by a Guthrie test carried out when the child is one week old. Treatment is by a special diet from which most of the usual proteins are excluded because of their phenylalanine content. If this is started early and rigorously adhered to, the child should develop normally. The children affected are often fair-haired and blue-eyed; if untreated their growth is stunted and they become physically retarded and severely mentally subnormal.

Brain Damage

Injury to a potentially normal brain may be incurred at birth, e.g. by anoxia or severe jaundice; or later as the result of meningitis, encephalitis, hypoglycaemia, severe dehydration, metallic poisoning or fractures of the skull.

EARLY SIGNS AND SYMPTOMS

Some of the clinical signs of specific conditions have already been described. Many babies appear normal until they start to fall behind in their physical development. Smiling is frequently delayed. These children are often poor feeders, making little effort to suck, and in due course resisting the introduction of solid foods. The general muscle tone is often low and they lie passively in their cots, taking little notice of their surroundings. Alternatively some are irritable and restless with a high-pitched cry which is difficult to calm.

Most subnormal children lag behind because they lack the drive and inquisitiveness to investigate and try out new channels of activity; thus they never experience those things normal to a child of their age and so they fall even further behind. As they get older they have a strong tendency to repeat the same action, or sound, or word, over and over again (perseveration). They dislike change and easily develop set patterns of behaviour which are hard to break, like sitting and rocking, or various mannerisms of the hands. Drooling is also common even when there appears to be no physical reason for it.

Initially it may be difficult to distinguish between mental and physical handicaps (cerebral palsy, deafness, defects of vision). An accurate diagnosis may only be possible after prolonged observation. Delay in social responses and motor behaviour and the exclusion of other handicaps indicates the likelihood of mental subnormality.

FITS

Fits are neither a cause nor a sign of subnormality but a great number of mentally subnormal children have fits of either the grand mal or petit mal variety. Although not causing subnormality in the first instance, continuing, uncontrolled fits can result in further cerebral deterioration. The most common drugs used to control fits are phenytoin and sodium valproate. Phenobarbitone is also often used but may cause hyperactive behaviour and further impair learning ability.

MANAGEMENT OF THE HANDICAPPED CHILD

As already stated all young handicapped children have much in common. For one reason or another they suffer from lack of opportunity to learn and develop in the same way as their normal brothers and sisters. They need help. This help may be initiated in treatment, but success or failure depends on how it is translated into the daily routine. Parents play the major part in this, for it is they who have to care for the child and teach him all the things learnt automatically by a normal baby. It can be a long and difficult task.

One must not forget that there are other family commitments. The parents may be stunned to find that they have a handicapped child. In view of this, it is necessary to consider what demands in the form of home treatment should be made. To start with it may be better to suggest the best way to do the things which have to be done, e.g. changing nappies, feeding, playing, sitting rather than to recommend 'exercises' which could well become an additional burden.

One of the most difficult things for parents to accept is the fact that it is often impossible to forecast how far their child will develop. It is also sometimes difficult to explain that although there is no cure for the basic condition it is still possible to help the child develop more fully by special attention to handling, play and management. Parents need the help of all members of the paediatric team, doctors, therapists and social workers, to achieve a realistic approach and to persevere in the training of their child. As members of the team, parents should be encouraged to contribute their own observations which may be surprisingly astute and much can be learned from listening to their comments. Advice should be given as soon as possible so that the months of infancy are not wasted.

One characteristic of mentally handicapped children is their difficulty in initiating any activity; they may have adequate sight, hearing and sensation, they may be able to move, but they cannot link the two. In treatment a way must be found to bridge the gap, to motivate and eventually teach independence. Another factor, following from lack of motivation is resistance to change. This is shared by many physically handicapped children who find it difficult to move and prefer to be left alone. It is essential that they should be moved so as to change their position and activities at regular intervals. It is also important to progress from one activity to the next as soon as the first is becoming established. A list of possible activities may be useful at home or if the child is in hospital so that nothing is forgotten.

As a normal baby learns from the people and things around him, it is important that the handicapped baby should have not less but more opportunities to learn in this way. Mothers (and fathers) are often afraid to disturb their baby because they know there is 'something wrong with him' and need to be reassured that he needs to be picked up and played with like any other baby. It is important to talk to these children even when they are too young to understand so that they become aware of the shades of expression in the voice and in the face. Talking also helps the mother to relax and thus makes a better relationship between her and her child.

Some subnormal children do not present for treatment until they are two years old or more, when they are placed in Special Care nurseries. The suggestions put forward may be adapted by therapists or nurses for use with these older children.

Early Play

For young babies and the severely retarded it is important to establish eye contact as the first step.

1) Mother should have the baby on her lap, and facing her; she should encourage him to look at her, to hold up his head and to look around. When he can look from side to side, he should learn to look up and then down.

2) The prone position can be introduced early, during bathing and dressing, when baby can lie across mother's knee for a few minutes; the time should gradually be extended so that he gets used to the

position and can enjoy looking at toys, or his brothers and sisters moving round the room.

3) The mother should make the child aware of his limbs by handling and moving his arms and legs; showing him his hands and feet, naming them and other parts of his face and body as she helps him touch them with his hands.

4) Games and rhymes such as Pat-a-cake, Peep-bo, This Little Pig Went To Market, etc. teach many things. They may be normal routine in some families but are unknown to others who have been deprived themselves in childhood, or who have a different cultural background.

5) A variety of colourful and different sounding toys, rattles and squeakers will stimulate interest and help to improve eye, head and hand control. Small toys should be placed in the child's hand. He may at first need help to shake a rattle but gradually the help can be withdrawn so that he does it himself. A favourite toy can be held to make him reach for it. Baby balls can be used to hold between his two hands in a similar fashion.

Although 'mother-play' (and 'father-play') are important it is necessary that the child has time and opportunity to play on his own. His cot should be provided with a play bar on which a selection of toys and rattles are suspended (Plate 18/1). These must be adjusted so they

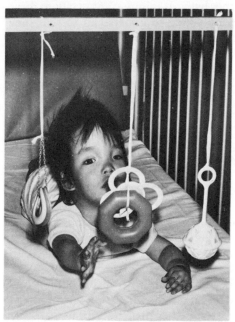

Plate 18/1 The 'play bar' in use in a hospital cot

Plate 18/2 Child lying over a
wedge pillow to encourage
head control while the hands
are free to play

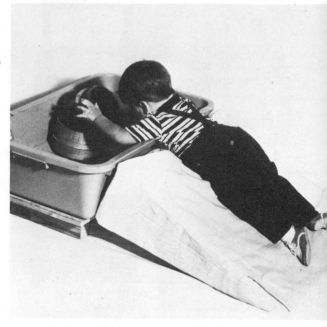

can be seen and touched. They should provide a variation of colour,
shape, sound and texture, and should be changed frequently.

FLOOR PLAY

All babies and physically retarded children should spend several
periods each day in the prone position. Older children who have not
done so may be quite helpless and miserable in this position which
they have never known. These children may find it more tolerable to
lie over a foam wedge which makes it easier for them to lift their hands
and to play with toys on the floor in front of them (Plate 18/2).

It may be difficult to convince the parents of the necessity for an
older child to play on the floor in this position, when he can appear
more socially acceptable propped in a chair. But floor play must
continue so as to develop movement and mobility. Rolling is important as an early form of mobility but other means of progression (on
knees, seat or feet) must be encouraged as an alternative. A tummy
trolley or Shasbah trolley (designed for spina bifida children) may be
appropriate for some children and enable them to explore their surroundings. Once able to move under their own volition they become
more interested and better motivated to do so.

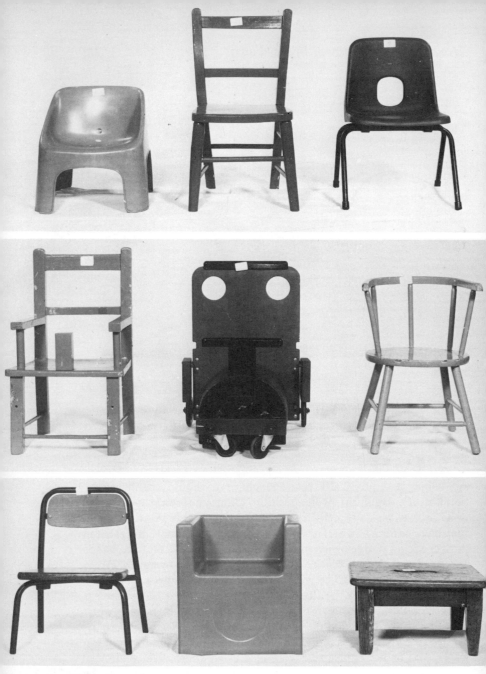

Plate 18/3 An assortment of seats demonstrating variety of height, width, shape and support. The selection of a seat is important, whether the handicap is minimal or severe. In general the feet should rest easily on the floor and the back or arms of the chair give adequate but not unnecessary support

Sitting

Sitting up is important for mental development and for the acquisition of head and trunk control. A suitable chair should be found quite early, and used for several short spells during the day. The selection of the chair demands careful assessment of the child's needs and abilities particularly if there is a physical handicap. Consideration must be given to fit, comfort and safety. The chair should be placed so that the child can watch what goes on, as well as being able to play with toys.

A cut out table with a built up rim will prevent toys falling off; they can be further secured by tying them with string through holes bored through the rim of the table.

The type of chair should be reviewed regularly with reference to the child's growth and physical progress. At first he may need full support. As soon as he acquires some head control he should sit for short periods in a chair only extending to shoulder level (Plate 18/5A); the first chair is then gradually withdrawn. Many types of chair are available, a wooden nursery chair can be adapted to many individual needs. Plates 18/3 and 4 show a selection of chairs.

Plate 18/4 A high-backed corner seat, made for a child with no head control. The tray is adjustable to different heights; the cushion is shaped to assist hip flexion and abduction. If required a foot rest can be fitted to the base which is on castors, and has a door stop brake either side so that it can be safely left in a ward or nursery among active children

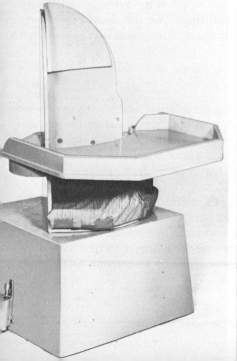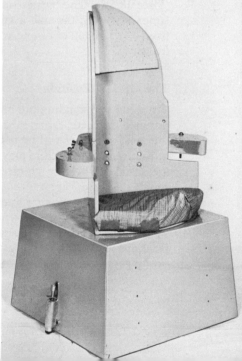

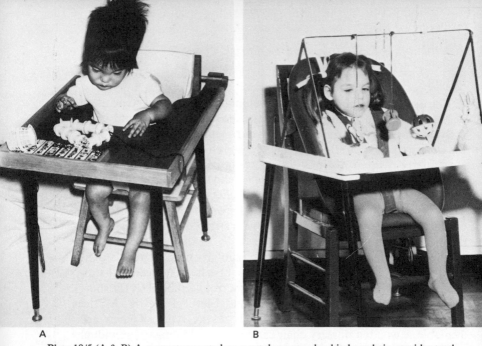

A   B

Plate 18/5 (A & B) A car seat mounted on a cut down wooden kitchen chair provides total support when head control is absent. An adapted nursery chair without head support should be introduced as soon as possible (18/5A). The cut out table with rim is essential. Plate 18/5B has an additional bar on which to hang toys at eye level

For the multiply handicapped child the Britax Star Rider car seat makes a useful first chair giving maximum support in a good posture (Plate 18/5B). The harness can be replaced by webbing and Velcro straps fastening through a central ring. The seat must be securely fixed on a kitchen or dining-room chair, or on a specially constructed frame.

The Upright Position

Kneeling and standing can be started relatively early so as to provide as much different experience as possible. Support from the physiotherapist or helper will be necessary at first. Both positions are best introduced with the child playing at a table of suitable height. If there are sufficient helpers children may benefit from playing together round the table.

Standing splints are sometimes useful for children waiting for calipers to be fitted, or for hypotonic or mentally subnormal children, so that they learn to appreciate some independence in the upright position (Fig. 18/1). In the latter case the splints are withdrawn when no longer needed. Splints can be made of Plastazote, Orthoplast,

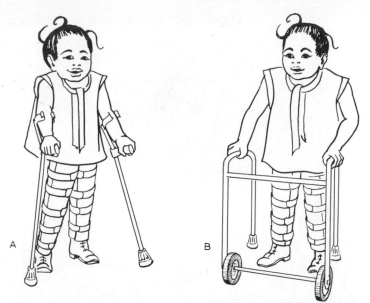

Fig. 18/1 Wearing canvas splints while awaiting calipers, progression to elbow crutches is easily achieved (A) after learning to walk with a Ripmaster walker (B).

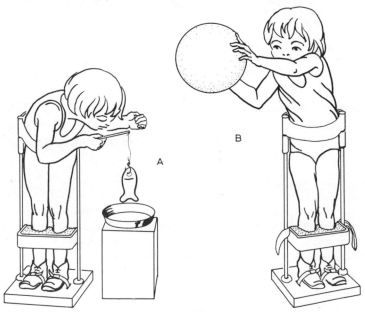

Fig. 18/2 The Flexistand or Newcommen Stander used to control pelvis and legs while the child enjoys games designed to encourage trunk rotation and co-ordination of the upper limbs

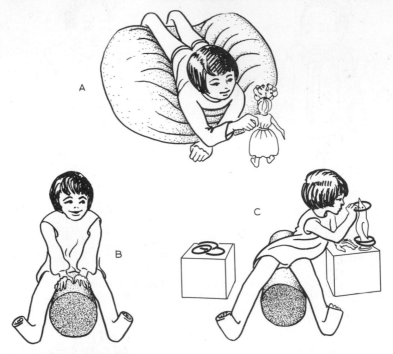

Fig. 18/3 Activities in bilateral above knee plasters: A. Lying prone over a sagbag is comfortable and fun. It can be started very early and encourages back extension; B. Long sitting on a roll is easier than on the floor; C. In this position balance and rotation are practised

plaster of Paris or of canvas, with steel supports and webbing and Velcro straps. The Flexistand or Newcommen Stander is also useful for some children; it can allow free movement of the upper part of the body (Fig. 18/2).

Treatment in Plaster

Many children require operations and spend long periods in plaster. This time should not be wasted. It can often be used to continue treatment and to make further progress. Much can be done to improve the function of other parts of the body (Fig. 18/3).

Walking

Baby walkers, the Cell Barnes walker and pushing toys are discussed on p. 243. Older children who can co-operate and whose arms are relatively unaffected may find the Rollator or the Ripmaster walkers more appropriate to their needs. Each has its advantages and disadvantages. The Ripmaster is less known and although more difficult to manoeuvre in a small space is good preparation for crutch walking as weight is taken through the arms in a similar position (Fig. 18/1).

Some multiply handicapped children will unfortunately never be able to stand and walk alone, but the difficulties of management will be greatly eased if they can be left to stand holding on, and walk with help. Although this appears to be more important when they are older and bigger, it is better to start when they are still young. Less disabled children enjoy all the normal nursery apparatus, and water play, painting, swings, slides and climbing frames, all of which provide an incentive to exercise and exploration. They also like moving to music and action songs; these can be used to help overcome any specific physical difficulties, but the greatest benefit is in learning to do things with others and become independent. These activities may appear closer to the work of the playleader or nursery teacher than the physiotherapist; the ideal situation is one in which the two work together.

SUPPLIERS OF GOOD TOYS

Educational Supply Association and Abbatt Toys
    P.O. Box 22 The Pinnacles
    Harlow
    Essex

Fisher Price Toys made by Mettoy Playcraft Ltd.
    14 Harlstone Road
    Northampton
and available in many good toy shops

James Galt & Co. Ltd.
    P.O. Box No. 2
    Cheadle
    Cheshire
and branches in large towns

Mothercare Shops in most big towns

Reeves & Sons
    Lincoln Road
    Enfield
    Middlesex

Thomas Hope Ltd.
St Philips Drive
Royton
Oldham
Lancashire

REFERENCES

Levitt, Sophie (1977). Cerebral Palsy. Chapter included in *Neurology for Physiotherapists* (Ed. J. Cash) 2nd edition. Faber and Faber.

Nettles, O. (1977). Spina Bifida. Chapter included in *Neurology for Physiotherapists* (Ed. J. Cash) 2nd edition. Faber and Faber.

Younghusband, E., Birchall, D., Davie, R. and Kellmer Pringle, M. L. (1970). *Living with Handicap*. National Bureau for Co-operation in Child Care, London.

BIBLIOGRAPHY

Arkwright, M. (1969). *The Frostig Approach: Guidelines for Teachers*. College of Special Education, London.

Armour, C. (1977). 'A Patient's View of Spina Bifida.' *Physiotherapy*, **63**, 7.

Bowley, A. H. and Gardner, L. (1972). *The Handicapped Child*, 3rd edition. Churchill Livingstone.

Bryce, Jennifer (1976). 'The Management of Spasticity in Children.' *Physiotherapy*, **62**, II.

Childs, V. (1977). 'Physiotherapy for Spina Bifida.' *Physiotherapy*, **63**, 7.

Dubowitz, V. (1969). *The Floppy Infant*. Clinics in Developmental Medicine No. 31. William Heinemann Medical Books.

Dubowitz, V. (1977). 'Analysis of Neuromuscular Disease.' *Physiotherapy*, **63**, 2.

Eckstein, H. B. (1977). 'Spina Bifida: the Overall Problem.' *Physiotherapy*, **63**, 6.

Finnie, N. R. (1974). *Handling the Young Cerebral Palsied Child at Home*, 2nd edition. William Heinemann Medical Books.

Gardner-Medwin, D. (1977). 'The Management of Muscular Dystrophy.' *Physiotherapy*, **63**, 2.

Griffiths, M. I. (1976). 'Development of Children with Down's Syndrome.' *Physiotherapy*, **62**, 1.

Grimley, A. and Gordon, M. (1974). 'Clumsiness and Perceptuo-motor Disorders in Children.' *Physiotherapy*, **60**, 10.

Grimley, A. and McKinley, I. (1977). *The Clumsy Child*. Association of Paediatric Chartered Physiotherapists.

Higgon, G. J. (1977). 'The Child with Spina Bifida in the Special School.' *Physiotherapy*, **63**, 7.

Hollis, Katy (1977). Progress to improved movement.

Hollis, Katy (1977). Progress to standing.

    Both booklets are obtainable from the Institute of Mental Subnormality, Wolverhampton Road, Kidderminster. DY10 3PP.

Kapila, L. (1977). 'Primary Treatment of Spina Bifida.' *Physiotherapy*, **63**, 6.
Kirman, B. H. (1977). 'General Aspects of Down's Syndrome.' *Physiotherapy*, **62**, 1.
Kirman, B. H. (1977). 'Treatment and Management of Children with Down's Syndrome.' *Physiotherapy*, **62**, 1.
Madden, B. K. (1977). 'Orthopaedic Aspects of Spina Bifida.' *Physiotherapy*, **63**, 6.
Norris, J. (1974). *Choosing Toys and Activities for Handicapped Children.* Noah's Ark Publications, Toy Libraries Association, London.
Polani, P. E. (1976). 'Causative Factors in Down's Syndrome.' *Physiotherapy*, **62**, 1.
Richardson, A. and Wisbeach, A. (1976). *I can use my hands.* Noah's Ark Publications, Toy Libraries Association, London.
Sheridan, M. (1977). *Spontaneous Play in Early Childhood.* N.F.E.R. Publishing Company.
York-Moore, R. (1976). 'Physiotherapy Management of Down's Syndrome.' *Physiotherapy*, **62**, 1.

ACKNOWLEDGEMENT

The author wishes to thank Dr. Richard West, M.D., M.B., B.S., M.R.C.P., D.C.H., Consultant Paediatrician, St. George's Hospital, London and Mr. Travis Perera, MCH. ORTH., F.R.C.S., Registrar, the Orthopaedic Department, St. George's Hospital, London, for their help in the revision of these chapters; she is also grateful to Miss Glenifer Hodges and Mr. K. Cook for the photographs.

Chapter 19

Skin Conditions

by D. CANEY, M.C.S.P., DIP.T.P.
revised by B. V. JONES, M.C.S.P., M.A., DIP.T.P.

Few patients are referred to physiotherapy departments for the treatment of skin disease. The range and efficacy of other methods of treatment (drugs and dressings) have reduced the need for physiotherapists to spend their time in treating these conditions. However, a small number of patients are still referred. This usually occurs where drug treatment alone has proved inadequate to alleviate the condition, or where drug treatment is more effective if combined with ultraviolet irradiation.

In order to treat these patients effectively, the physiotherapist needs to have an appreciation of the methods of treatment available to her and a knowledge of the skin conditions concerned. She should also appreciate that the skin is frequently a mirror of the mental state of the patient. As in all other conditions she should therefore treat the patient as a whole rather than confining her attention exclusively to a localised area.

METHODS OF TREATMENT

Relaxation

If the patient is being treated by tranquilliser drugs, instruction in relaxation techniques may be of great benefit as an adjunct to treatment. Many physicians now believe that the ability of the patient to relax without recourse to sedative drugs (which may become addictive) is of prime importance. Because of this more patients who find it difficult to relax may be referred for instruction in the future. Physiotherapists should ensure that they are skilled in communicating the art of relaxation and should use this in the treatment of skin conditions, if the condition is related to mental stress. Training in relaxation is also important where the skin condition causes itching, e.g. eczema. The patient's natural desire to scratch will cause further skin irritation and the ability to relax will be of great benefit in controlling this.

Ultraviolet Irradiation

The beneficial effect of natural sunlight and the improvement seen in many skin diseases during the summer months, is sufficient indication of the value of ultraviolet light. Physiotherapists have traditionally used artificial sources of ultraviolet rays in the treatment of skin diseases. Dosage can be varied from the sub-erythemal dose, that is, 75 per cent of a first degree (E1) erythema dose, through all the degrees of erythema according to the desired effect. In clinical practice the effect aimed for is most likely to be increased cell production leading to thickening of the skin, increased desquamation, increased blood supply to the skin or increased pigmentation. Irradiation of the whole body is said to have a tonic effect. The usefulness of ultraviolet irradiation on areas denuded of skin, e.g. infected wounds, is doubted by many. It seems to be more logical and effective to culture the bacteria and apply the appropriate antibiotic. However, in a few cases, use of the abiotic rays of the spectrum may be appropriate.

When applying treatment the most appropriate ultraviolet source must be used. Treatment given with an air-cooled source of ultraviolet may be either from a mercury vapour lamp or fluorescent tubes. The spectra of these differ. The mercury vapour lamp gives rays from 184·9nm to 390nm (1849 Å–3900 Å) while the fluorescent tube gives rays from 280nm to 390nm (2800 Å–3900 Å). Where an erythema reaction is desired, irradiation from a fluorescent source will probably be the best choice as there is a higher percentage of the longer wavelengths. The initial choice of source is important as the same lamp must be used at subsequent treatments.

DEFINITION

The nanometre is now the official Standard International Unit of wavelength and has replaced the Ångström.

1 Ångström   = one ten millionth of a millimetre.
1 nanometre = 10 Ångströms
1 nm   = 10 Å

Prefix nano
Symbol n

Heat

The physiotherapist may also find that the application of mild heat has beneficial effects in the treatment of localised skin infections, such as boils, carbuncles or infected wounds. Heat may be applied super-ficially using infra-red rays or more deeply by short wave diathermy or microwave diathermy. The rationale underlying the use of heat is that increased metabolic activity and increased blood supply will aid the local tissues to combat the infection. The heat should be directed to the area of blood supply rather than towards the infection, so that the rate of bacterial growth is not stimulated (for example, heat could be applied to the forearm in the case of an infection of the hand). This type of treatment should be given in association with localised and systemic antibiotics.

Cold

An effective erythema can be obtained by massaging the local area with an ice cube. This may be preferable to the use of dry heat and is useful in the treatment of an area of skin which threatens to break down into a pressure sore.

Tissue Mobilising Techniques

Where the skin condition has led to fibrosis and thickening of the tissues, with the possibility of contracture and deformity, the mobility of the tissues must be maintained, and deep localised massage, with active movements and possibly passive stretchings, may be appro-priate.

ASSESSMENT AND RECORDING

In this field no less than in other areas of physiotherapy, the prelim-inary assessment of the patient's condition is essential. Careful obser-vation of the affected skin area should be made and the extent, type and severity of the eruption should be noted. Standard diagrams of the anterior and posterior aspect of the body are useful, so that the affected areas can be outlined and the pre-treatment record kept with the patient's treatment card.

A careful scrutiny of the patient's notes will be made in order to determine relevant points in the history of the condition, especially so that the type of medicaments being given can be known. Some of these may be sensitisers, e.g. coal tar, which will alter the patient's reaction to ultraviolet radiation. The patient's skin reaction to sunlight should be tested if the treatment prescribed includes ultraviolet irradiation. The result of this test and the other findings should be carefully recorded on the patient's treatment card. A special note should be made concerning the extent of the area treated so that at subsequent treatments the possibility of overdose because of altered screening is avoided.

In the treatment of most skin conditions re-assessment of the affected area should be made at each attendance, and the treatment should be based on the findings. A careful recording of the day-to-day condition and the consequent modifications to treatment is therefore of prime importance. Objective evidence such as a tracing of a wound, or the extent of an active area of acne, should be recorded rather than subjective assessments such as 'patient improved'. The physiotherapist should be in a position to base her reports to the dermatologist on factual evidence rather than optimism.

SKIN CONDITIONS REFERRED FOR PHYSIOTHERAPY TREATMENT

Acne Vulgaris

This is a chronic inflammatory disease of the sebaceous glands. The condition most commonly affects those parts where the glands are large, i.e. the face, chest and upper back, and is seen in adolescents and young adults primarily, though very occasionally, the condition may persist into later life. The essential lesion of the condition is the blackhead, or comedo, a firm mass of keratin which blocks the follicular pore. This may cause inflammation of the surrounding tissues or it may become secondarily infected with eventual fibrous tissue formation and unsightly scarring.

In mild cases no treatment other than careful skin toilet is required. Severe cases respond well to a prolonged course of a tetracycline antibiotic. The few patients who are referred for physiotherapists to treat are those who have severe acne which is not responding well to other forms of therapy. The rationale underlying this referral is that cases of acne improve in the summer months and therefore ultraviolet irradiation from an artificial source can be used to supplement the effects of natural sunlight. Exceptions to this are patients who have fair or sensitive skins, as they are often made worse by local ultraviolet radiation.

The affected skin should be washed with soap and water prior to treatment and gently dried with a clean towel and then irradiated by an air-cooled mercury vapour lamp. A first degree erythema is given to improve the condition of the skin and this is repeated when the initial dose has died down. A first degree erythema is preferred to a second as the aim of the treatment is to stimulate skin metabolism rather than produce desquamation. The technique of ultraviolet irradiation will vary with the area being treated. The physiotherapist must ensure that her screening techniques are such that there is no possibility of 'overlap' dosage. In the interests of the patient it is as well to screen to the natural bony features of the body, such as the jaw line or the clavicular line. A more acceptable cosmetic effect can be obtained by allowing a natural fade-off of irradiation, but this can only be done where screening is not essential.

Psoriasis

This condition affects approximately one to two per cent of people with white skin. The cause is unknown but the abnormality results in unduly rapid cell division within the epidermis. Normally the cells reproduce at such a rate that the epidermal turnover takes approximately 28 days. In psoriasis the turnover rate is seven times as fast, i.e. every four days. The amount of skin area affected varies from trivial to extensive. Characteristically, initial lesions are on the extensor aspects of elbows and knees and in the scalp, or over the sacral area. Severe cases may have total skin involvement, although the face is usually spared. The condition appears to be adversely affected by mental stress, although the course of the condition is typically unpredictable and exacerbations cannot always be attributed to this factor.

The affected area shows a slightly raised red plaque, with a sharp margin between it and healthy skin. The plaque is surmounted by dry silvery grey scales. If the scales are removed the underlying skin bleeds easily.

Medical treatment for psoriasis is usually by the administration of local or, very occasionally, systemic agents which contain a toxic substance to slow down the rate of cell division. Where these fail, or in the case of a patient whose condition is becoming rapidly worse, admission to hospital may be advised. It is in the intensive treatment of patients with psoriasis that the physiotherapist is most likely to become involved. The usual treatment is a modification of the Ingram regime. The patient bathes first thing in the morning in a tar bath and scrubs off his psoriatic scales. He then attends the physiotherapy department for general ultraviolet irradiation from a fluorescent source. As the irradiation is given daily, no more than a first degree erythema should be achieved and some authorities believe that a sub-erythemal dose only should be given. The lesions are then covered with dithranol paste and with a suitable dressing until removal the next day prior to bathing. Removal of the paste can be facilitated by the use of liquid paraffin. This treatment is effective in nearly all cases though many relapse again.

P.U.V.A.

Ultraviolet light has been used in the treatment of psoriasis for many years using minimal erythema reaction in conjunction with various preparations. Recent developments in the treatment of this skin condition have changed the approach in the management of psoriasis. It has been found that irradiation by long wave ultraviolet rays plus the oral administration of psoralens inhibits epithelial D.N.A. synthesis. Psoralens (8-methoxypsoralen) given two hours before irradiation results in a photochemical reaction in which the psoralens bind to the D.N.A. thiamine bases. Psoralens can also intercalate with two base pairs and give interstrand cross linkages (Pathak and Kramer, 1969; Cole, 1970; Dall'Acqua, Marciani and Ciavatta, 1971), this inhibits D.N.A. synthesis and cell division.

SOURCE OF IRRADIATION

Special fluorescent tubes have been designed to produce wavelengths between 320nm and 390nm – the psoralens being activated by wavelengths of 365nm. These burners are housed in a hexagonal shaped cubicle and the patient stands inside the cubicle and receives a general irradiation. This new technique is called P.U.V.A. which stands for psoralens and long wave ultraviolet.

MEDICAL AND PHYSIOTHERAPY TREATMENT

Three, four or five tablets of 10mg each (the number prescribed depends on kg bodyweight), are taken two hours before irradiation. If, on evaluation, the patient complains of nausea, the tablets should be taken at 15 minute intervals. The treatment must be prescribed by a consultant or other competent doctor.

DURATION OF TREATMENT

This depends on the individual's reaction to ultraviolet light:
1. Red-headed people who freckle are started at five minutes and progress by one minute up to 15 minutes.
2. People who redden and then tan are started at six minutes and progress by two minutes up to 20 minutes.

3. People who tan but do not burn are started at seven minutes and progress by three minutes up to 25 minutes.

The purpose of the treatment is not to produce an erythema reaction: if one should occur a suitable interval must elapse to allow it to subside before further treatment is given. Attendances are therefore limited to twice a week and should be spaced so that any reaction from the previous time would have become apparent before the next irradiation. This regime takes about six to eight weeks but the actual duration of the treatment is variable and will alter according to the time it takes for the lesions to clear.

MAINTENANCE DOSAGE

Each individual patient will be assessed. A possible maintenance scheme might be:

Once a week for four treatments, then once a fortnight for four treatments, followed by once in three weeks for four treatments and finally once a month for four treatments. The patient stays at the interval necessary to control the psoriasis.

PRECAUTIONS

The patient must always wear a pair of goggles and if there is no psoriasis on the face, a towel should be used to completely cover the face. The physiotherapist should remain within calling distance. The patient is instructed to take off the towel and goggles and leave the cubicle should he feel faint and to call the physiotherapist immediately.

Alopecia Areata

This is a relatively common condition in which patches of baldness appear spontaneously. There is no evidence to suggest that any type of physiotherapy will increase the rate of regrowth of hair in the affected areas, although high frequency stimulation and ultraviolet irradiation have been tried. Complete recovery of the affected patches usually occurs but may take from three months to two years. If ultraviolet irradiation is requested, a second degree erythema should be given to the affected area of scalp after careful cleansing with spirit to remove grease. Subsequent treatment would be given when the erythema of the previous dose has died down. The new growth of hair frequently lacks pigment but this is gradually developed.

Vitiligo

This is a condition in which there is a patchy loss of melanin pigment-ation. Areas of the body show irregular patches of skin lacking in pigment. The cause of the condition is unknown but it is sufficiently widespread to affect one per cent of the population. Recent advances in the treatment of this condition have shown some success in re-pigmentation after treatment of the affected areas with trimethyl-psoralen lotion followed by exposure to sunlight. The drug should be applied to the skin or alternatively taken by mouth approximately two hours before ultraviolet irradiation. The dose should be sub-erythemal and repeated not more often than every five days. The course should be prolonged, extending over a period of three to four months. During this time the affected patches should show evidence of re-pigmentation. If there is no response in this time the treatment is discontinued. However, if improvement is occurring treatment is continued for many months. Unfortunately the re-pigmentation may not be permanent and relapses occur frequently.

SKIN INFECTIONS

Furuncle

A furuncle or boil is an acute staphylococcal infection of the hair follicle. The infection discharges through the hair follicle after a series of inflammatory changes in which necrotic tissue is broken down into liquid pus. Any area of the body can be the site for a boil but areas of friction such as the back of the neck are the most likely. A series of boils affecting different parts of the body is known as a furunculosis.

The patient is first aware of pain and an area of redness is visible over the site of the infection. This becomes a raised area which quickly shows a yellow centre. After a short while the skin over this central core breaks down and pus is discharged onto the surface. Frequently a solid core of unliquefied pus is also discharged. The affected area is quickly repaired by fibrous tissue and a scar is left to mark the place where the boil existed.

A single boil is very often left to run its own course. Patients who are obviously prone to this kind of skin infection may be treated with appropriate antibiotics, such as penicillin. Only a few patients will ever find their way to a physiotherapy department. The treatment for those who do will depend upon the stage in which the boil presents itself. In the early stage before the boil has started to discharge mild co-planar short wave diathermy should be given. This aims at provi-ding heat to the base of the boil, and the electrodes should be positioned so that the field passes deep to the boil. The treatment by heat accelerates the metabolic processes and encourages discharge of pus. Once discharge has occurred, the localised area may be treated by a more superficial type of heat such as infra-red radiation in order to aid the healing process. Boils which do not drain freely or do not discharge their contents completely may be treated by local ultraviolet irradiation using the sinus applicator.

Carbuncle

If the infection spreads subcutaneously to affect a group of hair follicles a large area of skin may break down to reveal a deep slough which may take a long time to heal. This kind of skin infection requires the administration of antibiotics. The patient may be referred to the physiotherapy department when the objects of physical treatment will be to aid the rapid breakdown of slough and assist in the healing of the affected area.

Treatment will be along the lines already indicated for a boil except that initially there is a wider breakdown of the skin and the area of infected tissue thus revealed should be treated by ultraviolet irradiation using a fourth degree erythema or double-fourth degree erythema to the affected area. The surrounding tissue should of course be carefully screened. Following irradiation the site may be dressed using a proteolytic enzyme such as Trypure. Both the irradiation and the enzyme will aid the breakdown of slough. When the area is clean the aim is to stimulate rapid re-epithelisation and this may be done by the administration of heat, or a first or second degree erythema dose of ultraviolet irradiation to the wound and surrounding area.

Hidradenitis Axillae

The apocrine sweat glands of the axilla are occasionally the site of a severe chronic bacterial infection which may be confused with furunculosis. The condition is more severe and may run a chronic course over 10 to 15 years, during which time there is severe scarring with possible contracture of the fibrous tissue.

The condition appears first as multiple red tender nodules which eventually break down and suppurate. Spread of infection occurs with increasing involvement of all the apocrine glands until these are ultimately destroyed.

Treatment is by local and systemic antibiotics and in order to encourage free drainage surgical interference may be necessary. Scrupulous cleanliness of the area is essential in order to combat the superficial spread of the infection. The patient may be referred to the physiotherapist for mild short wave diathermy to the axillary region in order to encourage the free evacuation of the infected material by the application of heat. It is also important to ensure that the patient understands the need to maintain a full active range of movement in the shoulder joint to prevent contracture of the axillary tissue.

Pressure Sores

A sore is a popular term for almost any lesion of the skin or mucous membrane. A local impairment of the circulation caused by sustained pressure can result in a pressure sore. The damage to the tissues is the result of a temporary reduction in the blood supply. The changes can be observed at various stages. At first the skin appears erythematous and it is important to note the colour changes as the part has a livid hue just before the skin breaks down. Once the skin has broken down it becomes an open wound which may easily become infected.

PREVENTION

In order to prevent the occurrence of pressure sores, patients who are immobile should be encouraged to relieve pressure from weight-bearing areas at frequent intervals either by moving themselves into a different position or, if they are in bed and immobile, they should be turned frequently. They may be nursed on medical sheepskins, ripple mattresses, sorbo packs or in a Roto-rest bed. Strict hygiene should be observed and local massage over the area of pressure may be carried out.

If the area shows signs of redness over the pressure area, frequent mild thermal doses of infra-red may be given to improve the circulation. In addition, massaging the local area with an ice cube may be performed.

SKIN BREAKDOWN

If the skin breaks down, a first degree erythema dose of ultraviolet using the longer wavelengths is given to stimulate growth and increase the skin resistance. The circulation is maintained by infra-red irradiation on alternate days. If the part becomes infected then stronger erythema reactions will be required to combat the infection by making use of the bactericidal effects of ultraviolet.

Infected Wounds

A wound is an injury to the body caused by physical means with disruption of the normal continuity of the body structures. An open wound is one that has a free outward opening. An open wound which has become infected may be treated with ultraviolet. The surrounding skin should be protected and a local irradiation given. The degree of erythema depends on the condition of the wound; if there is pus a fourth or double fourth dosage is used initially, and is reduced as the infection clears. As granulation tissue appears the dosage should be reduced to a third or second degree, possibly protecting the area of granulation or using a blue uviol filter or cellophane to filter out the shorter abiotic rays. The surrounding skin may be given a first degree erythema using the Kromayer lamp at a distance or an air-cooled mercury vapour lamp.

CLEANING AND DRESSING THE WOUND

The wound will need to be cleaned before treatment and afterwards dressed with the appropriate medication using a strict aseptic technique.

SINUSES

If there is a sinus involved then a suitable quartz applicator should be used with the Kromayer to enable healing of the sinus from below upwards.

PHYSIOTHERAPY AS AN AID TO DIAGNOSIS IN SKIN CONDITIONS

Occasionally physiotherapists are asked to assist in the diagnosis of skin conditions. By using a Wood's filter in association with a Kromayer ultraviolet light source, certain types of tinea of the scalp (ringworm) can be shown as a bright blue-green fluorescence. Similarly, erythrasma gives a coral red fluorescence. This condition usually affects the groins, toe webs and the perianal region.

Photosensitivity and photopatch testing are used in the diagnosis of conditions where the skin has become hypersensitive to light. Such conditions may arise as the result of systemic or local exposure to a sensitising substance. There is a wide range of possible sensitisers including drugs (sulphonamides, chlorpromazine, tetracycline), soaps, antiseptics, and silver and gold salts. In other cases no direct cause for the hypersensitivity can be found. Because the tests require the use of an ultraviolet light source, physiotherapists may be asked to assist with them. A Kromayer lamp with a filter of ordinary window glass is used for the test. This eliminates rays below 320nm (3200 Å).

The minimal erythema dose (MED) for the lamp without the filter is calculated using a normal skin.

Photopatch testing is carried out in the following way. Patch tests of the suspected sensitiser are applied to both sides of the back or other suitable skin surface (one side then acts as a control). The patches are removed and the skin cleaned after 24 hours. The control areas are then covered with black paper to obscure the light. The test areas are irradiated by the Kromayer lamp with the filter using the minimal erythema dose. The areas are inspected 24 hours later. A positive reaction is shown by a reproduction of the photo allergy and the sensitising substance can then be identified. A comparison with the control side will show the degree of photosensitivity.

REFERENCES

Cole, R. S. (1970). 'Light induced cross-linking of DNA in the presence of a furocoumarin (psoralen).' *Biochimica et Biophysica Acta*, **217**, 30.

Dall'Acqua, F., Marciani, S. and Ciavatta, L. (1971). 'Formation of inter-strand cross-linkings in the photoreactions between furocoumarins and DNA.' *Zeitschrift für Naturforschung (B)*, **26**, 561.

Pathak, M. A. and Kramer, D. M. (1969). 'Photosensitization of skin in vivo by furocoumarins (psoralens).' *Biochimica et Biophysica Acta*, **195**, 197.

BIBLIOGRAPHY

Epstein (1966). *Archives of Dermatology*, pp. 93–216.

Rook, A., Wilkinson, D. S. and Ebling, F. J. G. (1978). *Textbook of Dermatology*, 3rd edition. Blackwell Scientific Publications.

Sneddon, I. B. and Church, R. E. (1968). *Nursing Skin Diseases*. Edward Arnold.

Wilkinson, D. S. (1977). *The Nursing and Management of Skin Diseases*, 4th edition. Faber and Faber.

Chapter 20

Burns

by R. WOOTTON, M.C.S.P.
revised by S. BOARDMAN, M.C.S.P. and
P. M. WALKER, M.C.S.P.

The Skin and its Function

It should be remembered that the skin is not just a collection of epithelial cells, but a composite organ of epidermis and dermis.

The epidermis is stratified and made up of five layers of cells, the deepest of these, the stratum germinativum, being the cell-producing layer.

The dermis is made up of two layers. In the upper layer lie the capillary loops, the smallest lymphatics and nerve endings including touch corpuscles, while the deeper layer consists largely of bundles of fibrous tissue with an interlacing of elastic fibres, and this rests directly on the subcutaneous tissue. This latter consists of bundles of connective tissue between which fat cells lie. The glandular parts of some of the several glands and deep hair follicles lie in this area. This subcutaneous layer serves to support blood vessels, lymphatics and nerves and protects underlying structures (Fig. 20/1).

The skin is the largest organ of the body, representing about 16 per cent of the total weight of the normal adult. It has many functions, but the two most important, when considering extensive skin loss in burns, are protection against invasion by bacteria and prevention of fluid and protein loss from the body.

BURNS

Causes

Burns can be inflicted in many ways, but in each case they result from tissues being subjected to excessive heat.

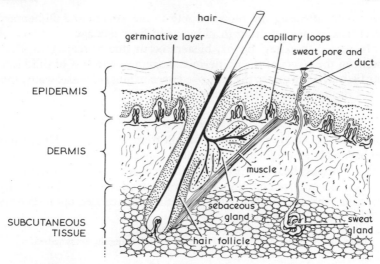

Fig. 20/1 A diagrammatic representation of the structure of the skin

Flame burns, scalds from steam or boiling water, contact burns or electrical burns, are the most common. Flash and chemical burns and indeed friction can all result in similar destruction and provide a Burns Unit with a great variety of cases from a wide cross-section of the population. Burns often result from accidents in the home, during work and play, and of course involve all age groups.

Effects

In any burn, particularly if it is extensive, the immediate and serious effects are shock, severe fluid and protein depletion, and the chance of gross infection if every possible care is not taken.

SHOCK

Shock is the first hazard to be combated or, better still, prevented. Crile has stated that 'the best treatment for shock is prevention' and since shock is anticipated in burns it can be counteracted by early treatment. In burns, shock is delayed and results from the fluid and protein loss from the blood due to the increased permeability of the vessel walls. Because of this loss, the viscosity of the blood is increased. The compound effect of decreased circulatory volume and increased viscosity leads to a fall in blood pressure based upon decreased venous return to the heart.

When fluid loss is allowed to continue vasoconstriction takes place, eventually affecting the blood supply to the viscera and alimentary tract, sometimes resulting in kidney and liver damage.

In partial thickness burns, blisters occur due to seepage of fluid between the layers of the epidermis. Together with loss of fluid into the tissues, again due to the increased permeability of vessel walls, this gives rise to gross oedema (Plate 20/1).

INFECTION

Infection is another serious complication in burns. Organisms embedded in hair follicles and sweat glands can survive the sterilising effect of excess heat and provide sources of infection. Further infection can occur from contamination from outside sources. This is why the isolation and treatment of these patients are carried out under the

Plate 20/1 A patient with a severely burned face showing the gross oedema

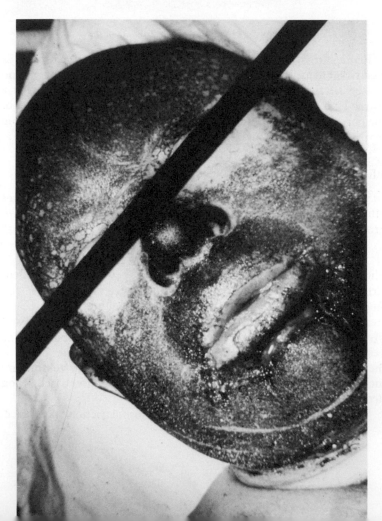

strictest conditions. The necrotic skin and constant oozing provide the ideal host for receiving and growth of bacteria, and where this is not adequately combated general toxic effects are produced. Local infection complicates surgery, for obviously where there is infection there will be an inability to accept grafts and consequent production of scar tissue.

Classification

Under this heading we must consider the depth, the size and the position of the burn in assessing its severity. Burns fall into two categories, partial thickness and full thickness. In the former, the epithelium and superficial layers of the dermis only are involved and healing can occur by first intention. In full thickness burns the dermis is totally destroyed and with it the epithelial lining of the sweat glands and hair follicles so that no regenerative islands are left and healing can occur only from the wound edges, resulting in unstable scarring and underlying contractures.

It must be borne in mind that the assessment of depth of some burns is not easily definable in the first 48 hours, and even then the difference between partial and full thickness burns can by no means be correctly defined. What appears to be deep may prove to be partial, and what is partial thickness may indeed become deep due to further destruction of partly damaged cells by pressure or infection.

Partial thickness burns may be acutely painful since the nerve endings are damaged, whereas in full thickness burns the nerve endings are totally destroyed, and therefore the acute pain and immediate systemic effects from it are often less severe. Burn areas, of course, are invariably of mixed partial and full thickness involvement.

The depth of the burn is dependent on the temperature to which the area is exposed and the duration of the exposure.

In assessing the extent of the area involved the 'rule of nine' is useful to remember (Fig. 20/2). The percentages of the total body area in adults are as follows:

head and neck	9%
front of trunk	18%
back of trunk	18%
arms	9% each
legs	18% each
perineum	1%

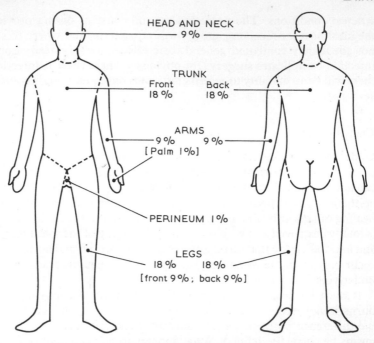

Fig. 20/2 The 'rule of nines' for assessing the extent of the burned area

It is of interest to note that the palm of the hand is 1 per cent. As a rule 20 per cent burns in adults and 15 per cent in children necessitate intravenous fluid replacement. No one area gives rise to greater fluid loss than another but it is stated that there is greater loss in superficial than in deep burns.

With regard to the position of burns, wherever hands, feet, face and joints are involved, these should be regarded as major burns. It is the obvious functional importance of hands and feet that place them in this category. Burns of the feet, because of their weight-bearing function, are major burns. It has been stated that the hands are, next to the brain, man's greatest asset and when they are burnt it must be remembered that man is robbed of a large quota of his independence.

Joints fall into this major burn concept because their flexor surfaces, so often involved, tend to contract, thus producing accompanying ligamentous tightening and if neglected, resultant joint changes. As far as the face is concerned, apart from the cosmetic importance of treating it as a major burn, burns of the eyelids can produce contracture. This in turn, because the result is inadequate coverage of the eyes, can lead to corneal ulceration. It must also be remembered that facial burns are often associated with inhalation burns and involvement of the respiratory tract, when tracheotomy may be necessary.

From the point of view of infection some areas are known to be much more prone to pseudomonas than others, e.g. the trunk and the inner side of the thighs.

The severity of burns is not estimated only by their extent, depth and position. The age and general condition of the patient must also be taken into consideration. The elderly and the very young are at much greater risk than other age groups, the former due often to their lower resistance to infection and their relative immobility resulting from possible secondary disability such as heart and lung conditions or arthritic joint changes. The more elderly the patient, the lower the percentage of burn that may prove fatal.

In children it is generally accepted that they are at great risk because the relationship between their total body surface and their circularised volume is such that they lose comparatively more essential constituents of the body through a burn of given extent than an adult.

General Treatment

The majority of severe burns are usually admitted to the casualty department of district general hospitals, where treatment should be commenced to provide:

1. An adequate airway
2. An intravenous drip
3. Suitable analgesia
4. Temporary dressings
5. Catheterisation

More and more specialised units are being established, and early transfer within the first 24 hours is ideal. These units provide the specialised care that is urgently required, and by their construction, equipment and management, are geared to minimise the chance of infection which is so very prevalent in burns. In most units patients are nursed in individual rooms where the temperature can be controlled and the patient receives all the intensive care that is necessary following such severe trauma.

At an early stage the airway should be checked. In cases of pulmonary complications endotracheal intubation or tracheostomy with pulmonary ventilation may be needed.

The replacement of fluid loss is of prime importance to counteract 'burns shock' but care is necessary to avoid under or over transfusion.

Urine output is carefully monitored and a urinary catheter allows hourly estimation.

Before the burns are dressed they are cleaned and the blisters are deroofed. Patients with superficial burns have them covered with porcine skin or paraffin gauze dressings, the former being changed every 48 hours but the latter left for one week. Deep dermal or full thickness burns are dressed with silver sulphadiazine, chlorhexidine or similar preparations; the dressings are changed every second or third day.

Superficial burns should heal by natural intent in about 12 days. Deep dermal and full thickness burns will require surgical intervention.

Over the years the time factor has been reduced for the excision of dead tissue, and in many cases the operation can be performed between two and five days after the initial burning. This is clearly beneficial as mobility and function may be quickly regained and the length of stay in hospital reduced. Where this is not possible because of the patient's general condition, surgery is delayed for three weeks during which time the slough will begin to separate. When patients sustain mixed thickness burns which are difficult to assess, dressings using silver sulphadiazine for three weeks are of infinite value, as they allow the depth of burn to declare itself. Any superficial and partial thickness burns will by this time have practically healed. When possible, the defect is covered by autografts, i.e. the patient's own skin.

The ideal environment for the treatment of burns is one where infection can be readily controlled. Patients are therefore isolated and this isolation can lead to difficulties in their management. Many patients suffering from burns find it depressing and frightening to be alone, and in some cases they may already have psychological and social problems, such as alcoholism, depression, or epilepsy; these problems need very careful assessment and treatment with the help of psychiatric and social workers. In making plans for future rehabilitation this aspect must not be disregarded.

In such an environment of isolation, treatment can be easily carried out, room temperatures can be controlled to individual needs and a strict aseptic routine can be followed at all times.

Ideally in the early stage, patients with extensive burns are nursed on low air loss beds (Plate 20/2). This is an air displacement system. The bed consists of five sections each adjusting to the body contour, the pressures of which can be individually controlled to suit the needs of the patient. Nursing care with this type of bed is simplified by:

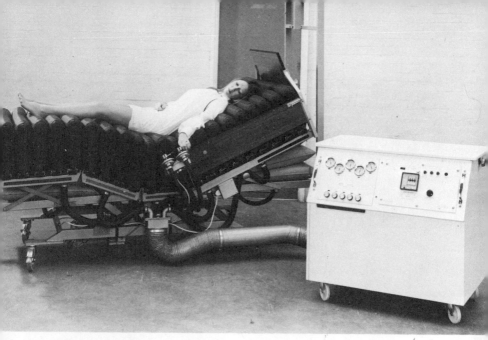

Plate 20/2 The low air loss bed

1. The elimination of pressure areas
2. Lifting and turning the patients is reduced to a minimum
3. Changing of bed linen is reduced as only a top sheet is required

Physiotherapists find that the tipping mechanism is easily controlled which is an asset in the treatment of the chest. However, they do criticise the fact that patients have difficulty in moving themselves around the bed and for this reason it is necessary to transfer the patient to a hospital type bed as soon as possible.

The hands should be elevated to prevent oedema and to prevent contractures hands are covered with silver sulphadiazine and placed in plastic bags or gauntlets so that exercises can be carried out easily and mobility maintained (see Fig. 20/3). The bags are changed daily or as required.

Saline baths used to be employed a great deal for the badly burned but in some units their popularity has waned, because of the dangers of cross-infection. However, when they are used, they can be invaluable in facilitating early movement and easing the removal of dressings. Patients can be immersed gently in tanks containing normal saline, diluted 1 in 20, at body temperature. The patient may be initially apprehensive but exercises under these conditions can be more comfortably carried out. These baths are given every two or three days and they are discontinued for at least five days after grafting. If the baths are not given, showers are of great value.

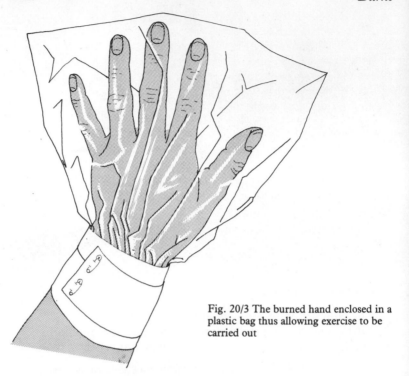

Fig. 20/3 The burned hand enclosed in a plastic bag thus allowing exercise to be carried out

Physiotherapy in the Treatment of Burns

Aims of treatment:

1. To prevent chest complications
2. To maintain mobility and prevent contractures

In extensively burned patients, breathing exercises are the earliest treatment given. Many of these patients suffer inhalation of hot and poisonous gases or steam, and the mucous membrane linings of the respiratory tract become inflamed and oedematous. Tracheostomy may have to be performed. This carries with it the danger of infection if it is not managed correctly. Suction should be carried out with the greatest possible care using a 'no-touch' technique. If the patient is ventilated, the physiotherapist may be asked to carry out vibrations while the doctor bag-squeezes, and the nurse uses suction.

After the patient has been extubated, an intermittent positive pressure breathing machine, such as the Bird or Bennett is often used. These machines are also of infinite value on patients who have an underlying chronic chest condition present prior to their burns.

It should be noted that children with burns of the face and trunk easily develop acute chest symptoms but respiratory complications often take 24 hours or more to develop.

If the patient has chest burns but no obvious respiratory complications, care must be taken; expansion only should be checked and vibration and percussions not given, as further trauma to already burned tissues may result in superficial burns becoming full thickness.

If burns are full thickness and circumferential, the patient will be encased in a tight armour of eschar (burns scab). The surgeon may perform a longitudinal incision or escharotomy in order to allow chest expansion and thereby prevent lung collapse.

Positioning of the patient is most important and a close watch must be kept on this by the physiotherapist as well as by the nursing staff. Burns overlying the flexor aspect of joints give rise to contracture. These must be prevented. Splints are ideal though with severe burns they are difficult to apply effectively. Plaster of Paris with Kramer wire, Plastazote, Polyform and Orthoplast are all used in an effort to support and maintain good functional positions of joints including the cervical spine. Here it must be stated that some contractures are not completely preventable, but it is still important that every effort is made to minimise them. The use of boards and splints to prevent foot drop are essential and knees should be maintained as straight as possible. The head and neck should be supported in a mid- and extended position. Since oedema is very prevalent in burns, hands in particular should be elevated by fixation to suitable apparatus beside and above the bed and sometimes upon well-placed pillows.

All movements can be encouraged from the time the patient is admitted to hospital. However, when autografts are applied, the grafted areas must not be mobilised for at least five days when the first dressing takes place. This does not prevent physiotherapists giving movements to ungrafted areas and it is indeed essential that they should continue them.

Movements can be commenced between five and seven days.

A feature of burns illness is a mental surrender to apathy – often aggravated by necessary isolation. Combined with this is a suppression of intellectual and aesthetic interests and a withdrawal from personal relationships. The physiotherapist's daily, or twice daily, visits give these patients a regular and closer contact with the outside world and this in turn demands of the physiotherapist a great understanding and the ability to provide mental stimulation. In some units complete isolation is maintained only during the pre-grafting period, then, after grafting, the patient is transferred to a three- or four-bedded ward where the encouragement and company of others is undoubtedly an added incentive to recovery.

The treatment of burns is extremely time-consuming for the physiotherapist. When burns are extensive it is necessary to encourage specific and general mobilisation and it must be remembered that these patients tire easily and must be allowed frequent rest periods. Time must be spent in encouragement, endeavouring to give confidence to patients who, due partly to their isolation and largely to the severity of their injuries, need maximum reassurance and come to look on their physiotherapist as a source of special contact with the rest of the medical team.

AMBULATION

This varies from unit to unit, but from the authors' experience it has been found that early ambulation is desirable. Red-line bandage or Tubigrip is used as support bandaging and patients with severe leg burns may also be walked before grafting.

It is advisable to swing the well-bandaged legs over the side of the bed before commencing weight-bearing. Following surgery, blistering of newly grafted areas can occur, due to the inadequacy of newly established circulation to the grafted areas and therefore weight-bearing may not commence for seven to ten days. Standing around is *not* permitted and when sitting out, the lower limbs should be elevated. Crêpe bandages, Tubigrip or elastic stockings will have to be worn for several weeks by those with grafted legs, to prevent oedema. The adapting of footwear may be necessary where there is need to compensate for contracture (e.g. tight calf contractures may need a heel-raise) or to relieve specific pressure areas. This can be done with foam rubber or Plastazote.

The patient should attend the physiotherapy department at the earliest possible opportunity and this is often the patient's first contact with the outside world following the burn. Here supportive therapy and great encouragement is required because the disfigurement caused by the burn is often demoralising. Helping patients to surmount and overcome their natural self-consciousness is something in which the physiotherapist can play a very helpful role.

THE HAND

The hand is a perfect piece of mechanism on which man is constantly dependent. As such it is considered necessary to dwell a little on its individual treatment.

Hands are common sites for burns, not only through direct

involvement, but also because they are so often used in a reflex action to protect the face. There are more dorsal than palmar burns, partly due to the thick palmar skin.

Once again the maintenance of a good functional position is essential. The wrist should be extended, the metacarpophalangeal joints flexed, the interphalangeal joints extended and the thumb in abduction and slight flexion. If the patient is unable to maintain full active movements, or is unco-operative, splinting may be applied, and thus

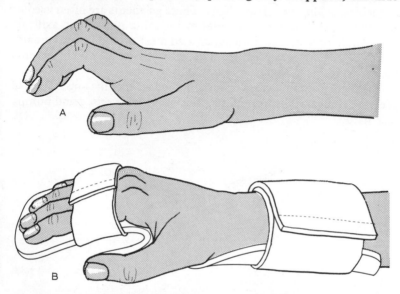

Fig. 20/4 A. The contractures of a burned hand; B. Corrected by adequate splinting

the typical burns deformity of the hand, i.e. dropped wrist, hyperextended metacarpophalangeal joints and flexed interphalangeal joints, is prevented (Fig. 20/4).

After healing, sensation is not entirely normal, and patients must be warned of the dangers of coming into contact with direct heat, i.e. hot plates, radiators, etc. as well as against exposure to sun for at least 12 months. Once the grafts are healed and skin becomes more stable, the patient attends the rehabilitation department where the physiotherapist gives the patient hand exercises. Warm water baths can also be of value but no direct heat in the form of infra-red lamps or wax should be given. Massage with hand cream such as lanolin is given in order to soften the scar. These treatments are usually carried out in conjunction with the occupational therapy department.

Advances originating in the U.S.A. are being made in the prevention of hypertrophic scars after burns. The method has been adopted in this country and is proving most successful. It consists of the use of precisely-measured pressure garments, such as gloves and stockings, made of an elasticated mesh material. The wearing of such garments can start at about two weeks after the burned or grafted areas are healed (Plate 20/3). It has been found necessary to insist on these being worn 24 hours a day for 6 to 18 months, except for brief periods to enable washing etc. (Plate 20/4). These garments are often used in conjunction with splints, the latter maintaining pressure in axilla or neck where pressure from the elasticated mesh would be inadequate. It is the exact and even pressure of these two materials which prevents the formation of disfiguring and disabling scars.

The theory of the success of such methods is that the application of pressure elongates the fibroblasts, thus preventing raised and bumpy scar tissue.

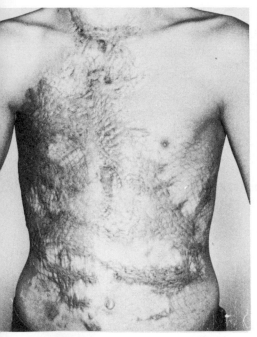

Plate 20/3 A patient with a healed burned and grafted chest

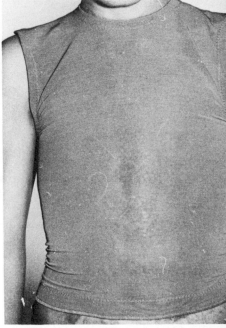

Plate 20/4 The same patient as in Plate 20/3 wearing a precisely measured pressure garment to prevent the development of hypertrophic scars

Watch must be retained over patients thus treated after their discharge until the pressure can be safely removed, i.e. until the hypertrophic tendencies are overcome.

Sometimes cortisone is injected into the scars.

METHODS OF SKIN TRANSFER

1. Free skin grafts which are without a blood supply for up to 48 hours after transfer
2. Skin flaps, which are joined to the body by a functioning arterial and venous flow

Free Skin Grafts

These are of two thicknesses.

SPLIT SKIN GRAFT

These can vary from the very thin to three-quarter skin thickness and are cut with a knife or dermatome. Such grafts are used very largely in the surgery of repair and particularly in the grafting of burns. After cutting, they are applied to the raw areas with a backing of Tulle Gras. The donor sites heal within 10 to 12 days.

The patient may be nursed exposed or with dressings, according to the wishes of the surgeon. The recipient area must always have a good blood supply and be free from necrotic tissue and infection, (particularly haemolytic streptococcus).

For the first 48 hours a split skin graft survives on the exudate from the underlying granulating tissue. By 48 hours capillaries will have grown into the graft and vascularised it. The formation of haematoma or tangential movement of the graft will prevent vascularisation and the graft will fail.

Following skin grafts, movements can be commenced after five to seven days. Joints not directly involved in grafting can be moved, but movement of these must not cause friction on the newly applied skin. Once the grafts are well-established, the application of a bland cream, e.g. lanolin, is desirable, to soften the scars. This should be gently kneaded in – 'heavy handedness' must be avoided, otherwise blistering occurs.

Full thickness burns require split skin grafting in order to gain a skin cover; however, this often contracts considerably and may either have to be replaced or released at a later stage with more split skin or full thickness grafts being added, or skin flaps used.

FULL THICKNESS GRAFTS (WOLFE GRAFTS)

These are small and of full thickness skin, excluding fat. They are usually taken from the post-auricular or supraclavicular area to repair facial defects such as eyelids. The donor site will not regenerate and must itself be closed by a split skin graft or direct suture.

In burns of the face, eyelids are often involved and since their contraction can lead to corneal ulceration it is important to apply a graft at the earliest opportunity. The Wolfe graft contracts less than a split skin graft and this is therefore the graft of choice.

Skin Flaps and Pedicles

Skin flaps and pedicles consist of skin and subcutaneous tissue.

They take their own blood supply and so can be used to graft over areas where the blood supply is poor or non-existent, such as over bone, cortical bone, joint cartilage and over bare tendon. Flaps do not contract so that they can be used to prevent or correct deformities. Transfer of skin flaps can sometimes only be done in stages so that the viability of the graft can be maintained. In some flaps there is a 'random' supply of blood vessels. Other flaps are designed to include at least one sizeable artery or vein. The latter type can be much longer.

The forehead, acromio-pectoral and deltopectoral flaps are the most used. The principal types of flaps are a) transposition flaps, b) pedicle flaps, c) direct flaps and more recently d) free flaps due to the advent of micro-surgery.

TRANSPOSITION FLAPS

These are used to replace defects by transposing skin and subcutaneous tissues from an adjacent site, such as might be employed in the grafting of pressure sores. These in themselves demand little from the physiotherapist.

PEDICLE FLAPS

Pedicle flaps are raised and sometimes tubed and are used most often for the replacement of traumatic defects of the face and neck. Indeed, in many units this type of graft is widely used as a means of conveying skin from one part of the body to another.

Nasal and chin defects are made good in several ways, but from the point of view of physiotherapy, the acromio-thoracic tube pedicle and the abdominal pedicle are important to mention, although nowadays they are less used. The acromio-thoracic pedicle is raised from the upper chest wall and the lower end is swung into position to repair the

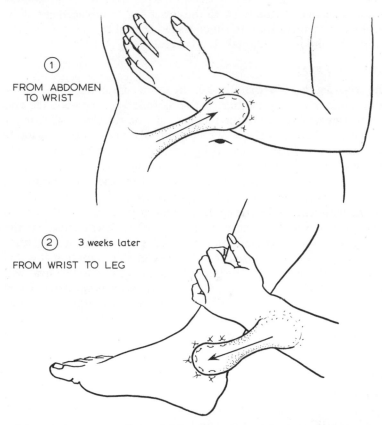

① FROM ABDOMEN TO WRIST

② 3 weeks later

FROM WRIST TO LEG

Fig. 20/5 (1) The abdominal pedicle is raised and attached to the wrist; (2) The abdominal pedicle end is detached and re-attached to the ankle area

nose or chin defect and then held in place for three weeks. This will necessitate a mild side-flexion and rotation of the neck. The abdominal pedicle is raised from the abdomen; one end being taken to the wrist and then in stages to the recipient site (Fig. 20/5).

DIRECT FLAPS

These are open, their under surface remaining raw throughout their attachment period.

Pedicle and direct flaps are both means of making good one area by robbing another. They can be transposed from one limb to another or via an intermediary, e.g. a flap or pedicle raised on the abdomen can be attached to the wrist, and after three weeks it is detached from its base and carried by the wrist to the lower leg as replacement skin. Un-united fractures are often encouraged to heal by the fact that the compound site is given good skin cover.

CROSS-LEG FLAPS

The cross-leg flap is perhaps one of the more common in use, one leg being the donor for the other. A flap is raised on the good leg and attached by its free end to the recipient site on the other. The donor site itself is then re-surfaced with a split skin graft. The position is maintained for three weeks during which time the physiotherapist supervises joint care and muscle function regularly. Some of these repairs entail most acrobatic positions and often lead to discomfort in the joints involved and to muscle spasm. Such tension and consequent pain may be relieved by the application of heat or ice and massage to the joints involved. Great care must be taken to prevent damage to the flap by heat, for the circulation is reduced and burning and destruction might ensue. There is also an absence of skin sensation and this must be remembered, for the patient, not being able to feel heat will therefore not be able to give any warning if it becomes excessive. Deep kneading of the muscles can relieve spasm and discomfort in a matter of a few days. Exercises in the form of static muscle contractions should be given and movements of joints where possible. Ice can also be used.

FREE FLAPS

This is a flap completely detached from the donor site and transposed directly to the recipient area. The blood vessels are dissected out – at least one artery and one vein – and anastomosed with vessels in the recipient area using an operating microscope.

This method of transferring a flap is of infinite value as there is no hindrance to movements as the donor and recipient sites are not attached to each other.

Following major burns, extensive rehabilitation is essential as scar tissue continues to contract for many months after the burn. This needs the co-operation of the whole team, including physiotherapist, occupational therapist, social worker and other medical staff. Consideration must be given to the type of aids, splints, etc. which the patient may require.

As many burns units cover a large area, the patients often live many miles away. It is essential, therefore, that good follow-up physiotherapy treatment is established in their local hospitals and the physiotherapists must make themselves responsible for setting up adequate lines of communication in order that the patient receives the best possible treatment.

BIBLIOGRAPHY

MacAllan, E. S. and Jackson, I. T. (1971). *Plastic Surgery and Burns Treatment*. William Heinemann Medical Books.
Muir, I. F. K. and Barclay, T. L. (1974). *Burns and Their Treatment*. Lloyd Luke (Medical Books) Ltd.

ACKNOWLEDGEMENT

The authors express their thanks to Mr. B. D. G. Morgan, M.B., B.S., F.R.C.S., Consultant Plastic Surgeon to University College Hospital, London, and Mount Vernon Hospital, Northwood, for his help and advice in the preparation of this chapter. They also thank Mediscus Products Ltd., of Wareham, Dorset, for providing Plate 20/2 showing the low air loss bed, and for their permission to reproduce it in this chapter. Finally they thank Mr. R. Blake, Sector Medical Photographer, Mount Vernon Hospital, Northwood, for help with the photographs.

Chapter 21

Terminal Care and the Physiotherapist

by P. A. DOWNIE, F.C.S.P.

With the increasing awareness of the needs of patients with progressive illness, and the advocacy of total care for the dying, physiotherapists are becoming more involved in these areas. For this reason
it seemed right to include a short general chapter on this aspect and to
indicate how physiotherapists may apply their skills for such patients.

We are constantly reminded that death is a taboo subject, but with
the increased number of special units being established for the care of
the dying, one might feel that the emphasis has now changed.
Elizabeth Kubler Ross in the U.S.A. has helped considerably in the
understanding of dying patients' feelings, as well as in the realisation
of the stages in bereavement; the work of Cicely Saunders towards the
understanding and alleviation of pain has revolutionised the basic
needs of many patients. Much of Kubler Ross's work can be classed as
commonsense and this is the prime requirement of the philosophy of
approach to the dying patient. While the stages which she describes
(Kubler Ross, 1970), are usually discussed in the context of bereavement it is interesting to see how they fit in with the reactions which a
person suffers when faced with disagreeable truths, e.g. the patient
who is told that he has multiple sclerosis, the mother who is told her
baby has spina bifida, the young man who has to be told that his leg
needs amputation after an accident. These stages can be summarised
as follows: denial of the fact, followed by anger and then the stage of
bargaining; depression follows and finally comes the stage of accep-
tance. Not every patient or family will react in the same way, nor will
they all go through each of the stages. If one understands that these
reactions are normal it will help the physiotherapist when she comes to
treat what to her may be considered 'a difficult patient'.

'Death is not merely an appendix to life in the manner of the ending
of a bad play that might turn out anyhow. Death is built into life's
structure and issues from its course. It is present long before the

conclusion, actually throughout the whole development of life. Life has been defined as a moment directed towards death' (Guardini, 1954). The care of the dying should therefore be seen as a part of the whole treatment plan for a patient. Certainly death is the last part of human life, but for everything alive it is this moment which is most crucial; death brings man's life to its fulfilment for good or ill and the shape of that life will require a conclusion to give it final validity. Death remains a reality but equally it does become a gateway into a new life. Within this truth there is a spirituality which can lift physical death to a higher plane and which gives the true purpose to life.

Care of the dying cannot be neatly slotted into a definite period of time; the actual process of dying may be sudden or it may be a progressive decline, of failing faculties and functions. It is about the latter group that most of the practical comments will be made, since it is these patients who require the encouragement and reassurance to accept their weaknesses and to live. It is of these that the question 'Should the patient be told of his approaching death?', will be asked. In general the answer is probably 'Yes', in as much as they are able to bear it. There is no need to be cold and dogmatic; rather sow the seed and then wait and see what follows. Certainly this telling should be done early in the care of patients so that they are able to assimilate the truth and to be helped to come to an understanding. Patients suffering from progressive disease, and particularly those who may have been treated with cytotoxic drugs, become less and less able to respond to the demands of brain and body and consequently, they look always to the familiar things.

Physiotherapy is not precribed because a patient is dying, but is an ongoing part of treatment that was started when the patient was more well. When I use the word physiotherapy I am thinking in the wide term of rehabilitation and total patient care. Some patients with a progressive disease, such as multiple sclerosis, motor neurone disease or severe arthritis, may have been in long-term hospitals for many years and received regular physiotherapy. To withdraw from treating such patients when they rapidly deteriorate would be most unkind, for this is the moment of truth when they require all the help that can be given. When one is privileged to partake in the work of any of the specialist homes for the dying, it becomes patently clear that the goal for each patient must be to live each day as it comes; for the physiotherapist this means adjusting the treatment each day.

Both doctor and physiotherapist, and, indeed, any member of the health care team, need to understand and appreciate the purpose behind treatment for the progressively ill or dying patient. Above all they need to accept that such care is as important as the care which they would bestow upon a young man who receives injuries in an industrial accident. Physiotherapy for the dying should not be regarded as a waste of a scarce professional's time. Death is neither a disaster nor a failure of medicine; but a natural event which terminates people's existence. Physiotherapy that helps the patient to accept his dying and eases his physical discomfort should be prescribed without hesitation.

Complicated treatments are not advocated, but with perception and adroitness it is possible to help many patients up to the point of death. There is no doubt that physiotherapy and occupational therapy have much to offer patients who are reaching the end of their lives. Active encouragement to continue to live each day will help the patient to a better adjustment of approaching death, and the mere fact that somebody is interested in a dying patient's whim or fancy can be therapeutic. For the paralysed and bedridden patient, passive and active assisted movements of limbs will help the circulation and ease uncomfortable joints. Massage has the dual advantage of physical help as well as providing an opportunity for the patient to talk. It needs to be continually repeated that the prerequisite in care of the dying is the ability to give time and to be able to listen and support. The role of the physiotherapist is essentially in this area.

Doctors do not prescribe physiotherapy because a patient is dying but if there is a mutual understanding between doctor and physiotherapist then he may well ask her to treat a dying patient that he may be enabled to die more peacefully. Into this category comes the progressively ill patient who develops pneumonia – 'the old man's friend' as Osler described it. Often, simple physiotherapeutic measures can relieve distress, and then it is justified; heroics in such cases are to be abhorred.

Relatives also need support. If the dying patient is being nursed at home, the visiting physiotherapist can help by showing the relatives how to offer unobtrusive help, how to move painful limbs and how to support where necessary as the patient potters round the room. This help with involvement in care will alleviate the feelings of inadequacy and despair which you so often encounter in families who are trying to cope and do not know how.

Dying patients latch on to unexpected things and people. The physiotherapist must be prepared for this and act accordingly. The author remembers a 60-year-old man who had been diagnosed as having a carcinoma of the bronchus for which no treatment was advised. He was admitted with an acute superimposed chest infection for which physiotherapy was requested. When seen he was acutely distressed and ill. Gentle breathing exercises and vibrations to the chest wall were instituted and with continuous oxygen he gradually relaxed and was able to co-operate. Over two or three days he improved, the infection cleared and he was mobilised to the point of going home. Suddenly his condition deteriorated and at the patient's request, the physiotherapist was sent for – in his own gasping words to the ward sister he said: 'She's the only one who's done anything for me.' When I reached him it was abundantly obvious that he was dying with no physical treatment being possible or justified; all I could do was to remain with his wife by the bedside. Care and compassion to the point of death must be accepted when one accepts the treatment of a patient with a progressive illness.

I have questioned whether physiotherapy should be prescribed when a patient is dying, but equally I ask the question, when is a patient dying? I remember a lady, aged 45, with disseminated carcinoma from a primary breast tumour. She developed 'pneumonia', and because the family could not cope was admitted to a nursing home for care and comfort. Twelve months later she was still in the nursing home being kept comfortable on opiates. It was decided to seek another opinion and she was re-assessed. Following this she was transferred for rehabilitation with a view to trying at home. She was weaned off drugs, mobilised, and a month later returned home where she remained for 18 months before dying.

Physiotherapy can also be used in helping nurses to handle patients with greater ease and comfort. Often the patient with advanced malignant disease may have bone metastases and nurses are afraid of handling limbs for fear they may fracture. Nothing transmits itself more readily than fear and if a nurse is afraid of handling such limbs, the patient will soon become aware of this. Firm gentle handling is necessary and often the presence of a physiotherapist, used to moving injured limbs, can give the required confidence to both nurse and patient alike.

The yardstick of all care of the dying is to improve the quality of life remaining in the individual patient; it may entail keeping one patient drowsy and thus unaware of pain, while allowing another patient to live more actively and even more dangerously than might normally have been considered (Graeme, 1975). A physiotherapist involved with care for a dying person needs to be able to appreciate the purpose of life as a whole; she must never be surprised by strange requests; she must certainly not attempt to impose her own ideas upon the patient; and her approach must be positive yet sympathetic.

PHILOSOPHICAL QUESTIONS

In these days of shorter working hours and great demands on the skills of physiotherapists, the question 'I have to treat dying patients and I cannot see the point – they won't recover and I could use the time more profitably' is frequently heard. Who are we to accept the truth of such a question? I would suggest that it is not for any one of us to say that a patient will not recover – very remarkable things do happen and I think it is right that we continue modified treatments, particularly for those patients whom we have known for a long time.

What do I say if a patient asks me if she/he is dying? At first sight, how difficult but most patients do not want an answer – that question is often the cry of desperation to be allowed to talk their way through their thoughts. Don't ignore it and don't run away. Rather sit down and listen, or, give some massage and listen, and turn the question to 'why are you asking me that' or 'what is it that makes you think this?' You will almost certainly find at the end that you have said almost nothing or you have been given time to provide the practical help required. Don't lie to such patients; if you don't know the answer, say no with complete frankness, *but* offer to either find out the answer or at least to find someone else who can help. In all these situations remember the hospital chaplain – he is there to help *you* as well as the patients.

'What do I do if I am asked to treat a dying patient for the very first time?' Here is another often asked question – particularly by students and newly qualified physiotherapists. Invariably it is asked in the context of the patient with disseminated cancer or some other progressive chronic disease, who develops a pneumonia. To any who postulate this question, I always say that if by treating such patients they will die more peacefully, then treat them; when in doubt in your own mind, ask yourself if you would allow your own parents to be treated – if you can honestly answer yes, then treat them. BUT, if you are unhappy about giving such treatments then you must say so. No one will think the less of you for so doing.

This chapter has not attempted to touch upon the problems of patients in intensive therapy units – it has concentrated on the patient who is dying from long-term illness. It is written to encourage the physiotherapist not to be frightened, put off or embarrassed at the thought of treating a dying patient. They are still human beings with all the faults and frailties which we know so well; they require help and if as physiotherapists we can provide this, then we must do so.

Certainly we may never know what our presence and actions have meant to the patient and the relatives; we ourselves will certainly learn how much the dying patient has given to us in the way of a better understanding of the total meaning of life.

REFERENCES

Graeme, P. D. (1975). *Support for the dying patient and his family*. Included in Proceedings of the Marie Curie Memorial Foundation's Symposium on Cancer, the Patient and the Family. John Sheratt and Son.
Guardini, R. (1954). *The Last Things*. Burns and Oates.
Kubler Ross, Elizabeth (1970). *On Death and Dying*. Tavistock Publications.

BIBLIOGRAPHY

Albanus (1978). 'to die or not to die.' *Therapy*, 5 May.
Downie, Patricia A. (1978). *Cancer Rehabilitation. An Introduction for Physiotherapists and the Allied Professions*. (Chapter 11.) Faber and Faber.
Hinton, J. (1967). *Dying*. Penguin Books.
Lamerton, R. (1973). *Care of the Dying*. Priory Press.
Parkes, Colin Murray (1972). *Bereavement*. Tavistock Publications.
Raven, Ronald W. (Ed. 1975). *The Dying Patient*. Pitman Medical.

List of Useful Organisations

Arthritis and Rheumatism Council for Research
Faraday House, 8–10 Charing Cross Road
London WC2H 0HN

Back Pain Association Limited
Grundy House, Somerset Road
Teddington, Middlesex TW11 8TD

British Rheumatism and Arthritis Association
6 Grosvenor Crescent
London SW1X 7ER

National Ankylosing Spondylitis Society
4 Beaconsfield Road
Clifton, Bristol

Disabled Living Foundation
346 Kensington High Street
London W14 2BD

Queen Elizabeth's Foundation for the Disabled
Leatherhead
Surrey KT22 0BN

Royal Association for Disability and Rehabilitation
25 Mortimer Street
London W1N 8AB

The Psoriasis Association
7 Milton Street
Northampton NN2 7JG

Association for Spina Bifida and Hydrocephalus
Tavistock House North, Tavistock Square
London WC1H 9HJ

Cystic Fibrosis Research Trust
5 Blyth Road, Bromley
Kent BR1 3RS

Down's Children's Association
Quinborne Centre, Ridgacre Road
Quinton Road
Birmingham B32 2TW

The Muscular Dystrophy Group of Great Britain
Nattrass House, 35 Macaulay Road
London SW4 0QP

National Society for Mentally Handicapped Children
Pembridge Hall, 17 Pembridge Square
London W2 4EP

Riding for the Disabled Association
National Agricultural Centre
Kenilworth
Warwickshire CV8 2LY

The Spastics Society
12 Park Crescent
London W1N 4EQ

Toy Libraries Association
Seabrook House, Wyllyotts Manor
Darkes Lane, Potters Bar
Herts EN6 2HL

Index